The Relaxed Patient

A Manual of Sedative Techniques

The
Relaxed Patient
A Manual of Sedative Techniques

GEORGE BAILENSON, D.D.S.

Adjunct Dental Anesthesiologist,
Department of Dental and Oral Surgery,
The Brookdale Hospital Medical Center,
Brooklyn, New York

Instructor, Department of Oral Surgery,
College of Dentistry, New York University

Fellow in General Anesthesia,
The American Dental Society of Anesthesiology

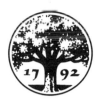

J. B. Lippincott Company
Philadelphia • Toronto

Distributed in Great Britain by
Blackwell Scientific Publications
Oxford and Edinburgh

I.S.B.N. 0-397-50292-3

Library of Congress Catalog Card Number 77-173257

Printed in the United States of America

1 3 5 4 2

Sharon, Thank You

Preface

This text is intended as an introduction to sedative management for practitioners in all fields of dentistry and presupposes no prior knowledge of these sedative modalities. Recognizing that more is required than a listing of suitable drugs, we have included clinically tested background on patient evaluation, treatment planning, monitoring of the patient's momentary status, modes of action of the various drugs and regimens, armamentarium and treatment of complications as well as basic cardiovascular and respiratory phenomena. (The inherent differences between sedation and general anesthesia are highlighted by a chapter on general anesthesia included to provide background and perspective rather than for implementation. General anesthetic management can be learned only by experience with a large number of cases in a supervised clinical situation.)

Following the progression outlined in the text, it should be possible for the general practitioner of dentistry as well as the specialist to start conservatively utilizing less critical techniques and to advance to more complex management using more potent methods and drugs for more profound effect. Because of the safety and simplicity of nitrous oxide analgesia, this modality serves as an ideal introduction to treatment of patients with altered consciousness, and has been so used for many years in our practice. Each technique presented is one in which the patient remains awake. Anesthetically speaking, this means that certain protective reflexes remain operative and with careful usage, safety should not be compromised. Gradually, using other agents and other routes of administration, the dentist can graduate to the use of a balanced medication utilizing combinations of methods and drugs, securing benefits here and avoiding disadvantages there.

Sedation techniques should be taught in the dental colleges and teaching hospitals where supervised clinical experience can be gained. Short courses in various sedative techniques are available in some areas independently of the dental schools. Ideally, in order to derive the greatest benefit from this text, it should be used to supplement such formal training. It is expected, however, that it would be used most often as the nucleus of a self-study program and, sensibly followed, should serve quite adequately in this regard.

GEORGE BAILENSON

The drugs here presented for use are relatively safe ones when used as directed (and allowing for some leeway), and were carefully selected as being unlikely to produce harmful effects. But because any drug can cause harm in certain situations or with certain patients, warnings against such possibilities are included. All reliable publications describing the use of drugs contain such listings of potential hazards.

Acknowledgements

Preparation of a text requires more than the desire to do so. It is imperative that the author possess a knowledge of the field and for this I am indebted to Joseph Turbin, M.D. for his tutelage, encouragement and assistance.

I wish to thank Donald Seuffert, D.D.S. for the techniques he suggested, Norman Amer, M.D. and Robert Taymor, M.D. for their review of portions of the text, David Brody, D.M.D. for his fine photographic work and Mrs. Joanne Pisano for her cooperation in posing for and expediting our photographic sessions.

In her various roles as sounding board, photographic model and typist, my wife, Sharon, has left her imprint indelibly upon this text. A task as large as preparation of a text requires many long hours of estrangement from one's family and these lost moments can never be recaptured. Only such an exceptional mate could have subordinated her understandable frustration with such a situation for the eventual benefits.

As an amateur author I could not have created this product without the guidance and cooperation of Mr. J. Stuart Freeman, Jr., Editor, Dental Books, J. B. Lippincott Company.

Contents

1 | Introduction

It is a relatively simple matter to numb any area of the mouth, and in most instances the effect can be reliably determined by objective signs; nevertheless, the dentist is often confronted by patients whom he cannot treat with comfort. Although actual somatic pain may have been eliminated, its psychological component has not.

Because of fear, emotional instability or various handicapping conditions, many patients are inadvertently denied optimal dental care. The treatment they do receive often falls short of meeting total dental needs and long-range maintenance of the oral apparatus in a condition of health.

Some persons are fortunate to have access to specialists who treat them with general anesthesia. However, the cost is high, such practitioners are unavailable in most locales, and the impersonal relationship inherent in infrequent treatment by a specialist militates against motivating these patients to accept dental care more willingly in the future.

The ideal situation would certainly be for treatment to be rendered by a dentist who has rapport with the patient on a continuing basis. Even if altered consciousness is mandatory, the patient should be familiar with the practitioner who would be better able to train and motivate him to accept dental treatment performed in a more normal fashion. A condition could be created that would predispose him to the best care and to periodic recall maintenance, the doctor's retention of the patient and attainment of optimal dental health.

Successful management of such patients requires an altered sensorium—sedation if you will—to lower their level of reflex irritability, thus allaying apprehension, promoting calm and facilitating subjective acceptance of the absence of pain. The number of persons for whom such methods fail is exceedingly small.

Consider also the patient who, through determination and perseverance, can allow himself to submit to dental treatment but whose limits are narrow. There are many procedures we perform today that require prolonged sessions whether they are part of an overall rehabilitative regimen or a single long appointment for some definitive procedure. These persons need help if they are to submit to this type of management. Unaided, they succumb to their nervousness, making care difficult and fatiguing for the dentist.

With techniques of modern medicine, there is a host of modalities available to dentists to further this aim. To begin a discussion of this nature, some definitions are helpful.

Simply stated, a *sedative* is a drug or agent that reduces functional activity of the central nervous system, producing a state of lessened excitation, agitation or reflex irritability, and depressed metabolic rate. A *hypnotic* produces loss of consciousness or a state of sleep. An *analgesic* relieves pain or lessens perception of pain sensation without loss of consciousness.

1

An *amnesic* obliterates memory. An *anesthetic* produces localized or total absence of sensation.

In clinical application, however, further detail and distinction are essential to comprehend these concepts of altered sensorium. Perhaps the key to understanding the ramifications in our dental situation can best be described as a function of the patient's awareness of his surroundings.

A well-sedated patient is somnolent in the absence of external stimuli but will react if they are applied. The so-called "protective reflexes" of the pharynx and larynx are operative; response to pain is present, although altered.

However, if the patient is maintained in a general anesthetic state, he displays no response to external stimuli and exhibits total lack of protective reflexes. Conduct of a case is vastly different, because vital functions, in the absence of sustaining mechanisms, must be assiduously monitored and managed.

Sedative medication requires concomitant use of analgesic or local anesthetic drugs. General anesthesia does not.

With sedation, amnesia is variable. It is usually present to some degree, but the amount varies from patient to patient and from one session to another for a given pharmacological regimen. Naturally, different agents or combinations of agents produce different results. With general anesthesia, amnesia is total.

In our dental situation where the operator usually functions both as surgeon and as anesthesiologist, sedative management is patently more expeditious. The simpler maintenance requires less attention and distracts less from the concentration necessitated by the operative procedures.

2 | Respiratory Anatomy and Physiology

Respiration provides oxygen for bodily function and eliminates the carbon dioxide waste production from the organism. The sequence includes the transport of atmospheric air to the lungs where oxygen diffuses into the bloodstream and is carried to the tissues for use in metabolic processes. Carbon dioxide, the main waste product of cellular metabolism, travels the reverse route from the tissues to the lungs for diffusion out of the blood and transportation back to the ambient atmosphere.

NORMAL FUNCTION

External Respiration

Conducting Portion

The airways of external respiration are, in effect, a connecting system of tubes that serve as a communication between the atmosphere and the lung alveoli, the site of actual gaseous exchange. The upper air passages include the nasal and oral cavities, the pharynx, the larynx, a cartilaginous structure which is divided by the vocal cords and leads to the trachea, a large, cartilage-reinforced tube passing down the neck anterior to the esophagus. The trachea divides into right and left major bronchi which, in turn, divide into many smaller bronchioles with fine lumens and thin walls, each leading to a single atrium with a cluster of alveolar sacs, the actual site of gaseous diffusion into the lung capillaries.

No diffusion occurs in this system of passages from the nose (or mouth) to the bronchioles and for this reason it is termed the *anatomic dead space*. The contained gases do no more than move in and out with each inspiratory or expiratory effort. Since the capacity of the system, approximating 1 ml. per pound of body weight or about 150 ml. for the average adult, does not change and the depth of respiration may vary; the resultant efficiency of inspiratory effort is subject to some variation. The first 150 ml. of air reaching the lung alveolar sacs comprises not fresh air but, rather, the contents of the passages with atmospheric air being drawn in only to the extent that the tidal volume exceeds the volume of the dead space.

Ventilating Portion

The diffusion portion of external respiration functions in the exchange of gases between the alveoli and the blood of the pulmonary circulation. The anatomy of this, the actual functional unit of the lung, consists of numerous lung alveoli, each supplied by a single bronchiole and separated from its investing capillary network by two thin endothelial membranes (the wall of the alveolus and the wall of each capillary).

Oxygen diffuses from the alveolus into the blood and carbon dioxide diffuses in the opposite direction according to pressure gradients determined by the partial pressures of the gases on each side of the membranes, the solu-

3

bility of the gases in blood and the physical properties of the membrane. Carbon dioxide is approximately 25 times more soluble in blood than oxygen and may diffuse more rapidly even in the presence of a lower pressure gradient. Disease processes in the lungs may alter the diffusion potential of the membrane. Pulmonary edema, for example, may lessen the amount of alveolar space available for gases and slow diffusion.

The term *physiological dead space* expands the concept of anatomic dead space to include all the air contained in alveoli that is not actually in contact with the epithelial walls. *Anesthetic dead space* goes one step further to include the dead space of the anesthetic equipment.

Internal Respiration

Transportation Portion

The transportation portion of the internal respiration carries the gases in the blood to the tissue cells. The pulmonary capillaries are oxygenated in the lungs and then introduce this oxygenated blood into the systemic vascular system. Carbon dioxide produced by cellular metabolism is returned by venous blood to the right atrium, then to the right ventricle and back to the lungs to be reconverted to arterial blood.

Most of the oxygen is transported by the blood combined chemically with hemoglobin in the form of oxyhemoglobin with only a small amount being carried in physical solution in the plasma.

Hemoglobin, a blood protein in the red cells, will combine with oxygen under certain conditions and release it under others according to the reversible reaction:

$$O_2 + Hb \rightleftharpoons HbO_2$$

The capability for oxygen saturation of hemoglobin varies as the oxygen partial pressure in the blood. The high oxygen concentration in the perialveolar capillaries promotes the tendency to combination with hemoglobin rather than release, as contrasted with the situation in the tissues where the relatively low oxygen tension favors its liberation.

Carbon dioxide is carried in the blood mainly as sodium bicarbonate in the plasma, but lesser amounts are transported either combined with hemoglobin in the form of carbaminohemoglobin, as carbonic acid in physical solution in plasma, or as potassium bicarbonate in the red blood cells. Normally, as much as 85 percent of the carbon dioxide is carried in the plasma.

Since venous pulmonary blood is characterized by an oxygen tension lower than that in alveolar air and a carbon dioxide tension which is higher, the pressure gradients favor diffusion of oxygen into the blood and of carbon dioxide out of the blood and into the alveoli for elimination. Since carbon dioxide in solution in the blood increases its acidity ($CO_2 + H_2O \rightleftharpoons H_2CO_3 \rightleftharpoons H^+ + HCO_3-$) through presence of hydrogen ions (carbonic acid) its diffusion out of the blood lowers acidity. The loss of carbon dioxide and lowered acidity enhances the affinity of hemoglobin for oxygen at the alveolar level.

Intracellular Respiration

Intracellular respiration involves the exchange of gases between the blood and the tissue cells. The culmination of the entire respiratory process is the delivery of oxygen to the cells and the removal of carbon dioxide. As elsewhere, the rate of interchange is regulated by the partial pressure difference of oxygen and carbon dioxide in the cells and blood. As tissue cells are more active, they deplete the local oxygen supply and accumulate carbon dioxide in the area. The reduced cellular oxygen tension causes more efficient withdrawal from the blood, and the higher cellular carbon dioxide tension favors more rapid diffusion into the blood.

INSPIRATORY AND EXPIRATORY DYNAMICS

Air enters and leaves the respiratory conduits as a result of variations in the internal pressure of the lungs caused by transient rhythmic alterations in the dimensions of the thoracic cavity. The chest cavity enlarges through outward and upward movement of the ribs on their cartilaginous connections and by the downward movement of the diaphragm. If these structures are mechanically unimpeded, free of disease and the airway is patent, changes in thoracic size will result in pressure variations within the lungs that will be equalized by inflow or outflow of air. In the normal resting phase between inspiration and expiration the lungs remain suspended within the thorax in a slightly stretched elastic condition, since some intrapleural, negative pressure always remains. If the chest wall is ruptured (pneumothorax) this slight residual negative pressure is lost, the lungs collapse because of inherent elastic recoil, and no air can be drawn in.

During a normal inspiratory sequence the thorax expands from downward movement of the diaphragm and an outward and upward movement of the rib cage which results from contraction of the intercostal muscles. Since the extrapulmonary areas of the thorax have no communication with the outside, no air can enter and thoracic cage expansion is accompanied by increased negative pressure. The lungs, surrounded by negative pressure, expand, thereby transiently increasing the intrapulmonic negative pressure until air rushes in (assuming a patent airway) to equalize internal and external pressures.

During expiration the sequence is reversed. Relaxation of the intercostal muscles and diaphragm causes the thoracic dimensions to become smaller. Increased intrathoracic pressure forces gas out of the lungs until, again, internal and external pressures are equalized.

Inspiration results from an active muscular effort. Expiration is a normally passive process brought about by the inherent elastic recoil of the thoracic structures but, in forced expiration, it can result from active contraction of the intercostal muscles.

Total lung capacity, in the average young adult male, approximates 6000 ml. but only about 450 to 500 ml., the *tidal volume*, moves with each usual inspiration or expiration. There are reserves so that more air can be brought into the lungs after the usual inspiratory effort, more can be breathed out after normal expiration. Even after maximal forced expiratory effort, about 1200 ml. of residual air remains.

In the normal conscious adult the respiratory rate falls in the range of 14 to 18 per minute while for children in the 60-pound range it is from about 22 to 26 per minute. Tidal volume in the same child would be about half the adult value of 450 to 500 ml.

REGULATION

The stimulus initiating respiration comes from the inspiratory portion of the respiratory center in the medulla. The expiratory portion of the same center acts in concert with the pneumotaxic center in the pons to inhibit the inspiratory stimulus, imparting a rhythmic pattern to respiration. Efferent impulses elicited by various reflex phenomena also cause cessation of inspiration and allow expiration to occur passively.

LUNG CAPACITY (YOUNG MALE ADULT)

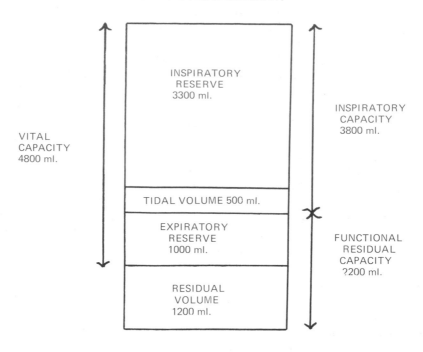

FIG. 1. Diagram showing the relative portions of the total lung capacity which are involved with each ventilatory exchange and those portions available as inspiratory and expiratory reserves.

The respiratory center acts as a clearinghouse, sorting out the various bits of information made available to it by afferent nerve impulses and directing appropriate responses through efferent nerve stimuli to effector organs. Basically, the phrenic nerve stimulates diaphragmatic activity and the intercostal nerves innervate the intercostal muscles and also some contributing abdominal muscles.

When the lungs are distended, stretch receptors in the alveoli are stimulated and the resulting afferent impulses to the brain, travelling along the vagus nerves, act to inhibit further inspiratory effort and allow expiration to occur. This reflex, the *Hering-Breuer reflex*, complements the activity of the

pneumotaxic center but is independent of it.

When oxygen is depleted in the blood, chemoreceptors located in the carotid and aortic bodies send respiratory stimulating impulses (primarily related to rate) to the respiratory center by way of the vagus and carotid sinus nerves. The *carotid and aortic body reflexes* (chemoreflexes) are activated by oxygen lack rather than by carbon dioxide accumulation (unlike the respiratory center) and may account for as much as 30 percent of normal respiratory urge. Oxygen lack, if it is severe enough, can render the inspiratory center inactive and, in this event, the chemoreflexes may remain as the sole stimulation of respiratory activity. Some of the barbiturates increase the sensitivity of this mechanism but nitrous oxide has no appreciable altering effect.

The *carotid and aortic sinus reflexes* (pressor-reflexes), activated by pressure on these structures, inhibit respiratory activity. The afferent nerves are the glossopharyngeal and vagus and efferent impulses travel along the vagi. Other neural mechanisms, arising anywhere in the body, may reflexly excite the respiratory center. These *peripheral or proprioceptive reflexes* may cause such effects as quickening of the rate due to powerful emotional experiences, increase depth of respiration during rigorous exercise, or cause a sudden gasp after perception of an unexpected severe pain.

The chemical makeup of the blood can affect the various neural determinants of respiratory function. Lowered carbon dioxide levels, by increasing the alkalinity of blood, activates chemoreceptors to augment both rate and amplitude of breathing.

The respiratory center, contrary to what might be expected, is only slightly affected by oxygen tension in the blood. Increased oxygen tension does not significantly slow respiration even though the need for further ventilation is lessened. Oxygen lack, particularly if the deficit is great, depresses the respiratory center. Carbon dioxide accumulation lowers the threshold of the respiratory center to reflex stimuli.

Voluntary Control of respiration, suspending or modifying the usual pattern, is possible, and without this potential one would be unable to talk, whistle, hum, blow, breathe deeply or hold his breath. Limits are imposed on this capability by chemical considerations but practice and training widen the range of voluntary control even as disease entities may narrow it. During consciously controlled respiration, impulses arriving at the respiratory center emanate from the motor cortex.

ANESTHETIC CONSIDERATIONS

Various premedicant agents and general anesthetics have the potential to depress the respiratory center and to alter the respiratory pattern. The patient must be carefully monitored for assurance that oxygenation is adequate.

Many of the classic signs of anesthesia relate to modifications of respiratory activity resulting from depression of the respiratory center by anesthetic agents. This is in addition to possible depression of the respiratory center caused by any hypoxia that may exist. Being less sensitive to carbon dioxide-induced stimulation, the depressed respiratory center transmits fewer and feebler impulses to the diaphragm and intercostal muscles with the possible result of decreased pulmonary ventilation. Insufficient ventilation can further result in hypoxemia and oxygen deprivation at the cellular level. If ventilation is seriously reduced (unlikely during sedative management) it should be assisted or augmented by manual compression of the reservoir bag.

Induction with inhalation agents depends on adequate alveolar concentration of the gas or vapor. If respiration is depressed, as may happen with overzealous premedication or sedation, unassisted breathing may be too shallow for uptake of sufficient agent to provide the desired hypnotic effect.

Certain physical factors affecting ventilation may also prevent adequate inhalation of agent. The trunk must be in such a position so as not to impede movement of the rib cage necessary for thoracic enlargement. The dead space of the anesthetic equipment should not be so great that, when added to existing physiological dead space, a lessened tidal volume cannot draw in sufficient fresh gas with each inspiratory effort. There should be no external pressure applied to the thorax or abdomen and the patency of the airway must not be compromised.

Airway obstruction is a constant possibility during general anesthesia (and, conceivably, during very deep sedation) but is of far less concern during light sedation (including analgesia). The most common causes of obstruction are faulty head position and changes in pharyngeal contour associated with jaw retrusion and a falling back of the tongue. If free exchange of gases is impeded, the chest wall will retract rather than expand during inspiration and a stertorous, or snoring, sound may be heard. Treatment consists of dorsal extension of the head and protrusion of the mandible by anteriorly directed pressure behind the gonial angles so that the jaw protrudes and the genioglossus muscle pulls the tongue forward. Pharyngeal airways, inserted either through the nose or mouth, will be tolerated by the patient only if he is sufficiently anesthetized for the gag reflex to be obtunded. Their use is not indicated during analgesia or moderate levels of sedation.

3 | Cardiovascular Anatomy and Physiology

The cardiovascular system provides both channels and propulsion for the transportation of blood throughout the body. The system delivers essential substances and removes metabolic waste products, as well as carrying the blood to and from the lungs for reconditioning by oxygen-carbon dioxide exchange. The heart, acting as a pump, supplies the propulsive force to the blood and the arterial system ramifies throughout the body leading into the capillary beds and terminates in the venous system where venules and veins consolidate to provide passage for the blood back to the heart and entrance once again into the cycle.

ANATOMY

Heart

The heart, with an intact septum partitioning the left and right sides, is actually two pumps. The left ventricle propels blood out to the systemic circulation while the right ventricle pumps its blood toward the lungs. The anatomy of both sides is basically similar as are their functions.

Chambers

The heart contains four chambers, an atrium and a ventricle on each side. Venous blood returns from the periphery and enters the right atrium through the openings of the vena cavae. It passes into the right ventricle and is pumped into the pulmonary circulation and on to the lungs. Reoxygenated blood returns from the lungs by way of the pulmonary veins to the left atrium and from here into the left ventricle which pumps it into the major artery, the aorta. The arterial tree branches through the body until the smaller arterioles are reached. These vessels terminate in a vast number of microscopic vessels, the capillaries, where the various exchanges with the tissue environment occur. Oxygen and various nutrient elements are given off and carbon dioxide and waste products are taken up. The blood enters a system of venules that grow to larger veins as they approach the heart.

Cardiac Muscle

Intermediate between skeletal muscle (striated and voluntary) and smooth muscle (nonstriated and involuntary), cardiac muscle is striated (both longitudinally and transversely) and involuntary. The heart must contract repeatedly for a lifetime and is not subject to only short periods of activity as is skeletal muscle. Further, it differs from skeletal muscle in its inability to metabolize anaerobically and in its incapability of developing a significant oxygen debt. Cardiac muscle oxidizes substrates very rapidly and, towards this end, is endowed with an exceptionally rich blood supply. Each cardiac muscle fiber has its own capillary, whereas in skeletal muscle the average is one capillary for each two muscle fibers.

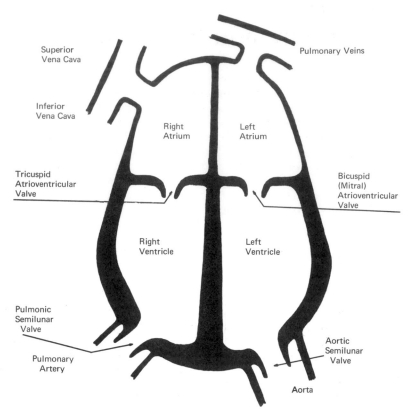

FIG. 2. Diagram representing the chambers of the heart, their valves and the vessels supplying and draining them.

The absolute refractory period for cardiac muscle fibers is longer than that for skeletal muscle. Cardiac muscle will not respond to a stimulus as long as the fibers are contracted. Since further contraction cannot be initiated until some relaxation has occurred, the sustained tetanic contraction of skeletal muscle is impossible.

Heart Wall

The walls of the heart are composed of three basic layers. The outer, the pericardium, is itself composed of two layers. The second (parietal) layer is fibrous, and the inner (visceral) layer is thin. Fluid between the two layers of the pericardium reduces friction that could be produced during movements of the heart.

The middle layer, the myocardium, is composed of interlocking muscle fibers, and it is this layer that supplies the contractile capability of the heart walls. The atria are required to do less forceful pumping than the ventricles and their myocardium is thinner. The left ventricle, opposing the greater peripheral resistance, must develop a mean pressure approximately seven times that of the right ventricle which pumps blood through a smaller, less resistive circuit. For this reason, the muscular development of the left ventricle is greater than that of the right and its walls are considerably thicker.

The inner layer, the endocardium, is formed by a smooth serous membrane that is continuous with the linings of the blood vessels and from which the heart valves derive their substance.

Heart Valves

Unidirectional flow of blood through the heart is achieved by the operation of a series of valves which close tightly during contraction and ejection and open during relaxation and cardiac filling. Each valve is comprised of two or three thin, flexible leaflets (cusps) composed of a small amount of fibrous tissue covered by endothelium. Forward-directed flow is not restricted by the valves but backward flow fills the cusps, causing them to close.

Regurgitation from the ventricles back to the atria during ventricular systole is prevented by the tricuspid atrioventricular valve on the right side of the heart and the bicuspid (mitral) atrioventricular valve on the left side. The three-cusped pulmonic semilunar valve guards against reflux from the pulmonary artery to the right ventricle and the aortic semilunar valve, also with three cusps, prevents backflow from the aorta to the left ventricle after ejection.

Divisions of Circulation

Systemic Circulation

The entire outflow from the left ventricle enters the aorta, the major artery of the body and one of great volume and distensibility. Its walls, which are thick and contain much elastic tissue, are designed to withstand the highest mean blood pressure in the body and, by distending, to accept the large bolus of ejected blood.

As blood travels farther from the heart it enters smaller arterial branches and some of its pressure head is spent countering resistance. As the vessels become smaller, they are required to contain lower pressures so that their walls can be thinner and contain less elastic tissue. In the arterioles the pressure is much lower and the elastic fibers are almost completely replaced by muscle fibers which can be stimulated to constrict the lumens, thereby regulating the flow to the capillary beds.

Capillaries, the smallest of the vessels, act as a bridge between the arterial and venous systems and it is through their walls (a single cell thick) that the exchange of substances between the blood and interstitial fluid is accomplished. This capillary wall diffusion is the basic *raison d'etre* for the entire circulatory system.

The number of capillaries in the body is tremendous, their total surface in an adult approaching 6300 square meters. Metabolically active tissues such as muscles and glands are more densely supplied with capillaries than are less active tissues such as cartilage or subcutaneous tissue. In all areas the capillary blood flow is regulated by variable constriction of the arterioles supplying them, and only a small percentage of the body's capillaries are open at any one time. This mechanism shunts blood to the areas where there is the greatest relative need at any given moment.

After traversing the capillary beds, blood is drained into venules and progresses through a series of ever larger veins until it, again, reaches the heart. In the venous tree the blood pressure is sufficiently reduced so that forward movement is not assured. Stagnation, pooling and backflow in these thin-walled vessels is prevented by the presence of numerous valves arising from foldings of the innermost layer of the vein walls.

Pulmonary Circulation

With each heart contraction a quantity of venous (oxygen-depleted) blood is ejected from the right ventricle into the pulmonary arteries to begin a relatively short journey to the lungs where it is converted to arterial (highly oxygenated) blood. The volume of blood expelled from both sides of the heart is equal but the pulmonary circulation contains only about 10 percent of the total blood volume, since its circulation time is only about 11 seconds as compared to more than a minute for the systemic circulation.

The pulmonary arteries proceed to the lungs where each one branches extensively. An arteriole is associated with each bronchiole and a dense capillary plexus surrounds each alveolus. Gaseous diffusion between blood and alveolar air is facilitated by this intimate relationship. The newly oxygenated arterial blood passes back to the left atrium to begin its circuit through the systemic circulation.

Coronary Circulation

Actually a division of the systemic circulation, the coronary circulation supplies the heart muscle itself. From an opening in the aorta just past the attachment of the aortic semilunar valve, the coronary circulation diverts approximately 5 percent of the total cardiac output through the coronary arteries, the very first branches of the arterial tree. Truly effective inflow occurs only during the ventricular filling and relaxation phase when the semilunar valve is closed.

The myocardium of the right atrium and ventricle is supplied by branches of the right coronary artery, and a similar arrangement exists on the left side. Each muscle fiber has its own capillary (as opposed to two fibers per capillary in skeletal muscle). After traversing the capillaries, blood is drained by coronary veins and reenters the right atrium by way of the coronary sinus and a number of smaller veins of Thebesius.

Abrupt occlusion of a coronary artery can lead to ischemia of the area of myocardium served by it. Necrosis and fibrosis of this area can occur and lead to impairment of cardiac function. Myocardial ischemia, when it occurs, is usually associated with substernal pain (angina pectoris).

Cerebral Circulation

The site of action of sedative drugs is brain tissue; the drugs are carried there by blood traveling in the cerebral circulation, a separate portion of the systemic system. Since these vessels are enclosed within the rigid cranium and incompressible and nondistensible structures, it is exceedingly important that arterial inflow be closely matched to venous outflow. Unlike other tissues where there can be variance in flow, the volume of blood within the cerebral vessels is relatively constant and the rate of flow must be regulated within a fairly narrow range.

Of all the body tissues, brain is the least tolerant of ischemia. Unconsciousness results from interruption of flow for as short a time as five seconds, and after only a few minutes irreversible damage occurs.

Cerebral blood flow is controlled by reflex mechanisms originating in the brain but affecting systemic hemodynamics as well as by local conditions. The main driving force of cerebral flow is the systemic arterial blood pressure and if this falls or rises, cerebral flow will increase or lessen in a parallel fashion. A second factor contributing to flow rate, the resistance of the vessels, is basically under autonomic control; but its effects remain within limits imposed by the systemic blood pressure. Vagal impulses result in dilation of the vessels, and sympathetic stimulation causes vasoconstriction. With a systolic blood pressure drop to 60 mm. Hg. adequate compensation is impossible and syncope results.

Carbon dioxide accumulation with its increased acidity will induce arteriolar dilation by direct effect on smooth muscle in the vessel walls. Epinephrine constricts cerebral vessels, but vasodilator drugs as well as intellectual activity, apprehension, emotional discharge, natural sleep and temperature changes do not significantly alter cerebral blood flow or oxygen consumption.

FUNCTION

Cardiac Cycle

With each beat of the heart a sequence of events is repeated—the heart fills, contracts, ejects blood and relaxes in preparation for the next repetition of the cycle. Both sides of the heart act in unison.

As ventricular contraction (systole) terminates, the atrioventricular valves are closed and the semilunar valves are open. The ventricular myocardium relaxes isometrically (no change in volume) and the intraventricular pressure drops sharply. The semilunar valves close because the pressures in the aorta and pulmonary artery now become higher than those in the ventricles, and the atrioventricular valves open. Blood returning from the periphery and the lungs enters the atria and can pass through the open atrioventricular valves into the ventricles. A major portion of the ventricular filling occurs immediately after the atrioventricular valves open but the rate of filling gradually decreases as the intraventricular pressure rises. Ventricular filling is completed with atrial systole as the atrial myocardium contracts in a peristalsis-like wave, each atrium transferring its blood to the ventricle ahead of it.

The atrial myocardium relaxes after its systole is completed, and with the drop in atrial pressure below that of the ventricles, the atrioventricular valves close. The fibers of the ventricular myocardium begin to contract. Since the ventricle is now a sealed chamber and since blood is incompressible, the ventricular pressure increases. During this time blood has been gradually leaving the aorta for the periphery and the pulmonary arteries for the lungs so that their internal pressures have been declining. When the building up of ventricular pressures exceeds that of the aorta and pulmonary artery, the semilunar valves open and a quantity of blood is rapidly ejected. As the ejection progresses its rate diminishes until pressures are equalized and the ventricle again begins its relaxation (diastole) and the cycle is repeated.

The intermittent pumping of the heart is converted to the relatively continuous flow of peripheral vessels by virtue of the elastic properties of the walls of the aorta and the major arteries. As the stroke volume is received into these vessels their lumens distend. Blood is always leaving the major arteries and in the interval before the next ventricular ejection, as the outflow proceeds (opposed, and somewhat regulated, by the arterial resistance), the vessels' return to their predistended state occurs as a result of the inherent elastic recoil of their walls. The arterial pressure varies somewhat about a mean and the limits of these variations, which can be measured with a sphygmomanometer, are referred to as systolic (highest) and diastolic (lowest) pressures.

On an average, approximately 70 ml. of blood is ejected during each systole by each side of a normal adult heart. Some residual blood remains in the heart after each systole, serving as a reservoir to help meet altered demands. In a failing heart, the residual volume may exceed the stroke volume.

Heart Sounds

When the heart valves close, they do so sharply and the ensuing vibration produces sounds that can be heard through a stethoscope applied to the chest wall. The first sound, heard upon closure of the atrioventricular valves, is the longer, softer and lower pitched of the two. Closure of the pulmonic and aortic semilunar valves produces a second sound which is higher pitched, sharper and of shorter duration. The sounds are classically described as sounding like "lub-dub," the "lub" spoken slowly and the "dub" terminating sharply. If the sounds are not short and distinct, this constitutes a diagnostic suggestion that perhaps the valves are not functioning properly.

Rhythmicity

Cardiac muscle throughout the heart exhibits the property of rhythmicity or the ability to initiate its own beat intrinsically and independently of intact nervous pathways. If the heart could be removed from the body without damage and with an intact blood supply it should, theoretically, continue to beat. The major role of the nervous system is to regulate the frequency and amplitude of contractions rather than to initiate them. Beats will begin only when some relaxation has occurred since the last contraction. This relatively long absolute refractory period prevents tetanization of the myocardium (which could prove lethal) and ensures that some filling will occur between contractions.

Conductivity

Impulses originate in the area possessing the greatest rhythmicity, and in the normal heart this is the sino-atrial (SA) node (pacemaker) located in the muscle of the right atrium near the opening of the superior vena cava. From here the cardiac impulse spreads as a wave of depolarization throughout the atria along ordinary atrial myocardial fibers until it reaches the atrioventricular node on the right side of the interatrial septum.

Passage of the impulse across the atrioventricular septum proceeds from the atrioventricular node solely by way of specialized conducting tissue, the atrioventricular bundle of His. In the course of this passage a slight delay occurs, and this is desirable because it allows for optimal filling of the ventricles during atrial contraction and because it prevents excessively frequent impulses of supraventricular origin from causing the ventricles to contract prematurely before adequate filling (possibly lessening cardiac output). A possible disadvantage of this single route of atrioventricular transmission is that if it is blocked atrial excitations may not reach the ventricles at all or may not reach them often enough to ensure adequate cardiac output. Atrioventricular conduction block can occur in inflammatory conditions (acute rheumatic fever) or as a result of drugs (digitalis).

After traversing the atrioventricular septum the bundle of His continues down the right side of the interventricular septum and divides into right and left bundle branches. The right bundle branch travels down the right side of the septum and the left branch passes through the septum and continues on its left side. Finally, the bundle branches give rise to the Purkinje system of conducting fibers that spread in a dense network over the walls of the ventricles. This very profuse ramification of conducting fibers causes almost simultaneous contraction of the

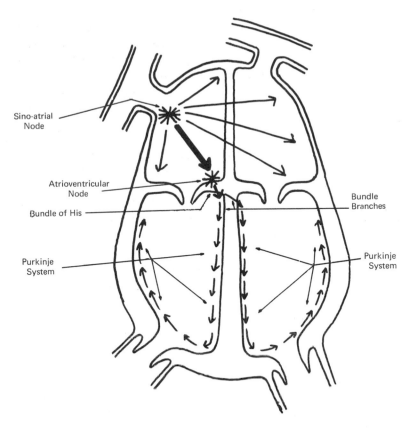

Fig. 3. Diagram representing the normal conduction system of the heart. Impulses originating at the sino-atrial node spread through the atrial walls and pass through the atrioventricular node and bundle of His to the Purkinje system of fibers in the walls of the ventricles.

entire ventricular walls as contrasted to the peristalsis-like wave of contraction characteristic of the atria.

All areas of the heart muscle possess rhythmicity but the sino-atrial node acts as the pacemaker because its rhythmicity is greatest. If the rhythmicity is diminished at the sino-atrial node or is enhanced at some other site, another region will take over as an ectopic pacemaker (focus). In descending order of rhythmicity, the areas likely to function as ectopic foci are the atrioventricular conducting tissue, the atrial myocardium and the ventricular myocardium. Impulses originating at any of these sites will not be conducted in the proper manner and cardiac function will suffer. If the atrioventricular conduction is completely blocked, the ventricles will beat at their own inherent rate (35 per min.) in complete lack of synchrony with atrial contraction, and cardiac output will be likewise diminished.

Regulation of Cardiovascular Function

Heart

The inherent rhythmicity of the heart maintains normal functioning potential but the frequency of the beats and the volume ejected per contraction are altered to meet changing requirements of the body by nervous, physical, chemical and mechanical factors. These changing conditions may represent physiological influences (exercise, digestion, sleep, emotion) or pathological (fever, hemorrhage). The normal adult heart rate of approximately 70 beats per minute (faster in children) is slowed during sleep and accelerates with muscular activity or emotional excitement.

Nervous regulation of the heart, primarily autonomic, is mediated by an accelerator center (sympathetic) in the fourth ventricle of the brain and a cardio-inhibitory center (parasympathetic) in the medulla. Some psychic control emanates from the cortex.

Sympathetic augmentor nerves from the spinal cord in the upper thoracic and cervical segments pass on the right side to the sino-atrial node to stimulate acceleration and on the left to the atrioventricular node and bundle of His for enhanced contractility. The heart rate is increased mostly by shortening the systolic phase; ventricular relaxation occurs more rapidly so that filling is enhanced; conduction is improved so that ventricular contraction is more synchronous and greater pressure is generated, and the coronary vessels dilate to meet increased demands of the myocardium.

Parasympathetic cardio-inhibitory fibers pass through the right vagus nerve to the sino-atrial node and through the left vagus to the atrioventricular conduction tissue. Parasympathetic influences depress the function of the pacemaker, the myocardium and the conductile tissue by antagonizing the augmentor influence of sympathetic nervous excitation. The heart rate slows (diastole lengthens) and decreased conductivity causes less powerful contractions.

Various reflexes, integrated in cardiac centers of the brain, act to maintain homeostasis in heart function. The *Bainbridge reflex* causes increased heart rate after stretch stimulation of vagal receptors beneath the endothelium and in the walls of the major veins brought about by increased venous return. *Pain fibers* in somatic nerves cause acceleration of heart beat. *Vagal afferents* produce a pressor response after a fall in blood pressure or a depressor response after a rise. *Baroreceptors* in the carotid sinus and aortic arch provoke a depressor response if the blood pressure rises and a pressor response if it falls. A *chemoreceptor reflex*, initiated by peripheral sensory receptors, primarily slows the heart by inhibiting the sino-atrial node and partially blocking atrioventricular conduction and secondarily will accelerate the heart, since concomitant stimulation of respiration and enhanced venous return overcome the primary reaction to chemoreceptor stimulation.

Physicochemical factors affect heart function. Elevated temperature, increased alkalinity and sodium and calcium in the blood accelerate the heart and strengthen contraction while acidity and excess potassium ions favor relaxation and lessen contractile strength. With exercise, increased carbon dioxide level and hydrogen ion concentration in the blood result in increased cardiac output, favoring filling by increasing extensibility of cardiac muscle and relaxing the heart. Mild hypoxia favors greater heart effort while severe hypoxia depresses cardiac function as it depresses the central nervous system. Asphyxia (high carbon dioxide and oxygen depletion) initially slows the heart but, as the condition becomes severe, increases the rate as the heart progresses to failure.

The adrenal medulla, acting as a component of the autonomic nervous system, secretes the catecholamines epinephrine and norepinephrine with a sympathomimetic effect on the heart. Adrenal cortical hormones augment cardiac function. Thyroid hormones make the heart more sensitive to catecholamines so that in hyperthyroidism the sympathetic nervous system is more active and the heart beats faster and more strongly and produces a greater stroke volume; it is more disposed to arrhythmias. Hypothyroidism produces the opposite result.

Cardiac output varies directly as does venous inflow. As ventricular filling increases, the myocardial fibers contract from a greater length, contractile force is augmented and the cardiac output increases.

Blood Vessels

Tissues differ in their need for blood according to their basal metabolic levels and according to the manner in which their metabolic rate is altered by the momentary state of activity. Mechanisms for regulation of flow are required, and these may involve neural mechanisms (skin, viscera) or local environmental conditions (heart, brain).

When a tissue is quiescent, its capillary beds close down and blood flow is shifted to other areas where the capillaries are open to receive it. Capillary flow is secondary to arteriolar regulation accomplished by constriction or dilation of the lumens of these vessels. Arteriole walls are composed chiefly of smooth muscle fibers arranged in circular fashion so that their contraction produces vasoconstriction and their relaxation results in vasodilation.

Generally, sympathetic adrenergic fibers (analogous to the cardiac accelerators) produce constriction, and parasympathetic fibers (analogous to cardiac inhibitors) dilation. There are also some cholinergic sympathetic dilator fibers originating in the cerebral cortex that pass to vessels in skeletal muscle. It is these nerve fibers that, when stimulated by apprehension or excitement, increased the blood flow to skeletal muscles in anticipation of increased exertion.

Locally, carbon dioxide excess and oxygen lack stimulate constriction and acids and metabolites lessen vascular tone resulting in dilation. Reaction to the presence of hormones varies but epinephrine and thyroxin are notable as vasoconstrictors.

The coronary vessels respond to autonomic innervation with the sympathetic nerves (which increase coronary flow) predominating; the vagal parasympathetic fibers have relatively little effect. Oxygen lack and certain drugs (epinephrine, xanthines) dilate coronary vessels and increase flow.

Since coronary inflow occurs mainly during diastole when the aortic semilunar valve is closed, there is less flow as the heart accelerates since systole accounts for a relatively greater portion of the cardiac cycle. However, as the heart works harder the increase in myocardial metabolism may dilate the coronary vessels to such a degree that this will overcome the curtailment of inflow time and the net result may be increased coronary flow.

Relationship Between Cardiac Output and Venous Return

Cardiac output and venous return are interdependent because, since the circulatory system is a closed circuit, the heart must pump all the blood it receives and cannot pump any not delivered to it. The major driving force propelling blood around the vascular circuit is the pumping of the heart which makes the blood go to areas of lower pressure. Exceptionally strong ventricular contraction may temporarily result in more blood in the arterial side than in the venous tree so that venous return is lessened and less blood is available to the heart; but over a period of time this will be equalized and venous return will match cardiac output. There are homeostatic mechanisms that regulate further ventricular function and peripheral resistance to achieve this end.

In the venous portion of the system, vessel walls are more distensible and blood pressure is lower so that pooling of blood is more likely to occur. This is countered by the presence of valves in the veins to prevent backflow. Muscular massage during activity squeezes the veins and, since the valvular arrangement permits flow in only one direction, blood will advance toward the heart. Without this arrangement blood would tend to pool in the lower trunk and legs when the individual stands erect.

Respiratory activity assists in assuring adequate venous return. During inspiration, the reduced intrathoracic pressure is reflected in lowered pressure within the blood vessels contained therein so that the venous pressure gradient becomes steeper and venous return accelerates. When the diaphragm descends during inspiration the resulting abdominal compression assists in this steepening of the pressure gradient. Expiration, with its increased intrathoracic pressure, tends to resist venous return but the effect is lessened by the action of the venous valves.

The ability of the heart to increase its stroke volume from a resting normal of 70 ml. to a maximum of approximately double that figure during extreme exercise depends upon adequate venous return. Augmented depth and rate of respiration as well as increased muscular contraction during exercise aid in maintaining this adequacy of venous return.

ANESTHETIC CONSIDERATIONS

In an anesthetized person the mechanisms maintaining venous return are depressed. Muscle tone that normally produces a milking action on vein walls is lacking. Respiratory function that normally aids venous return may be depressed. Anesthetic drugs may exert a direct depressant effect on myocardial contractility. Autonomic vasopressor activity that normally maintains capillary tone may be diminished.

Circulatory function should be closely monitored, and unnecessary anesthetic depth should be avoided. Maintaining the patient in a horizontal supine position favors circulation but may impede respiration because the abdominal viscera press against the underside of the diaphragm. The dental contour chair offers what may be the best compromise position for the patient. With the head on the same level as the feet, circulation will fare as in the fully horizontal position, and with the trunk in approximately a 10° upright position, the abdominal contents tend to fall away from the diaphragm.

4 | Patient Evaluation

Formulation of a dental treatment plan must include consideration not only of oral diseases or deficiencies but also a determination as to whether the proposed regimen is consistent with the general health status of the patient. As has been said so many times, we treat not only the teeth but also the entire patient. When medication is given for systemic effect, the medical evaluation becomes ever more critical.

HISTORY

It is our function as dentists to gather information and form an impression of the patient's tolerance for our procedures. We are not required to make definitive diagnoses and should not treat underlying systemic conditions. If there is any question as to safety or suitability of a given regimen, medical consultation should be sought. If any treatment is indicated, the patient should be referred to his physician.

This does not mean that the dentist's role is secondary in importance to that of the physician's. The dentist is the expert in his field (and should consult on that basis) but his area of expertise is oral medicine rather than general medicine. The final decision to treat, not to treat or to modify the treatment plan should be made by the dentist who has completed his diagnostic procedures after gathering information from all relevant sources (including the physician) and after he has determined the course of treatment including the methods to be pursued by or in conjunction with other specialists.

A new patient is an unknown quantity and we must learn as much as possible about him. Toward this end we use all our senses, plus intuition—acquired on the basis of many previous interviews with other patients and the experience gained from them. We extend the capabilities of our natural faculties with various mechanical diagnostic aids such as X-ray, thermometer, stethoscope, and sphygmomanometer, as the occasion may require.

QUESTIONNAIRE

One good source of information is the patient himself and, in the interests of conserving time, a method commonly used to narrow our range of questioning or direct its course is to ask the patient to fill out a medical history questionnaire. In addition to questions intended to establish the identity, occupation and financial responsibility of the patient, the questioning should include:

What is the reason for this visit?

Have you been under the care of a physician in the past 2 years?

Have you taken any medication regularly during the past 2 years?

Have you been in a hospital in the past 2 years?

Are you allergic or have you had any reaction to any foods or medications? Which ones?

Do you bleed excessively or bruise easily?

Have you gained or lost a lot of weight in the past 2 years?

Are you pregnant?

Do you frequently feel pains in your chest?

19

Do you become excessively fatigued when climbing stairs or walking fast?

Do your ankles swell during the day?

Do you often experience shortness of breath?

Do you sleep with more than 1 pillow?

Do you sweat excessively?

Do you have frequent dizzy spells?

Do you void frequently?

Are you often thirsty?

Do you smoke? How much?

Do you use alcohol frequently? How much?

Do you have frequent coughing spells?

Have you recently experienced any marked changes in taste, hearing or vision?

Have you ever had heart trouble, rheumatic fever, heart murmur, ulcer, persistent headaches, fainting, hepatitis, mononucleosis, glaucoma, prostate disease, asthma, bronchitis, anemia, tuberculosis, arthritis, jaundice, diabetes, goiter, tumors, cancer, sinus trouble, menstrual problems, stroke, high blood pressure, low blood pressure?

Have you ever been anesthetized?

Have you had any previous bad experience with dental treatment?

Have you ever fainted in a dental office?

OBSERVATION

Having secured a completed questionnaire from the patient, the interview should be continued by the doctor rather than the office nurse or receptionist, for several reasons. First, direct observation of the patient may suggest clues to the trained observer; second, a professional background may be necessary to evaluate equivocal answers; third, the doctor is best able to determine which areas of questioning to pursue.

The patient should be asked to describe the reason (chief complaint) for his coming to a doctor and this should be taken down in the patient's own words. A misunderstanding may be avoided at some future date if there is a record of the chief complaint as actually presented by the patient. Only when this is completed should you record your evaluation of the patient's complaint.

An alert questioner can gain much information by casual observation of the patient during the interview and by noting his physical constitution, gait, alertness, complexion, facial expression, speech, general level of intelligence and cooperativeness. Is the patient well-groomed? Does he wring his hands nervously? Is he irritable or depressed? Does his breath smell of alcohol or the ketones of diabetes? Are there numerous needle puncture scars along the course of the veins in his arms? Does his breathing sound labored? Does his intelligence seem subnormal? Does he recall facts, correlate thoughts and express himself well? What is his knowledge of dentistry? Is he submitting irrationally to a fear of infection, infirmity, cancer or pain?

An enlarged head may result from hydrocephaly, acromegaly or Paget's disease. Facial edema is a symptom of kidney disease, cirrhosis, angioneurotic edema, increased venous pressure or corticosteroid therapy. If a moon face is accompanied by hirsuitism and a buffalo hump back enlarged between the shoulder blades, suspect a Cushingoid syndrome from pituitary basophilism. Facial paralysis may result from a neurological disorder. A characteristic, dry, scaly, red-butterfly rash across the bridge of the nose is characteristic of lupus erythematosus, a collagen disease requiring the same prophylactic measures as rheumatic fever. Small lumps in the external ear (tophi) may be pathognomonic of gout. Saddle nose with notched incisors and mulberry molars (Hutchinson's triad) suggest congenital syphilis. Rose-purple cheeks with baglike swellings under the eyes and broad, coarse features may result from hypothyroidism (myxedema). Open mouth, thick lips, pinched nostrils, narrow dental arch, protruding teeth and mouth breathing suggest chronic adenoidal hypertrophy. Protruding, irregular, poorly calcified teeth associated with a receding chin can mean a history of rickets.

A wide-eyed staring expression with bilateral protruding eyeballs and exposed sclera suggests exophthalmic goiter (hyperthyroidsm); while unilateral exophthalmos can result from an inflammatory or neoplastic lesion of the affected orbit. The pupils may be constricted as a result of narcotic poisoning or old age, dilated because of belladonna drugs, deficient vision or strong emotion, or may be unequal due to a lesion of the central nervous system. The conjuctivae can be pallid with anemia or jaundiced from liver disease. Edema of the eyelids (especially the lower lid) can result from nephritis, anemia, or angioncurotic edema. Dark circles under the eyes suggest, possibly, lack of sleep, malnutrition or menstruation.

The tongue can be pallid in anemia, red or cyanosed in polycythemia, or deep, beefy red from vitamin deficiency. The papillae may atrophy in pernicious anemia, and the entire tongue may be enlarged as a result of cretinism, myxedema or mongolism.

Enlargement of the neck anteriorly (particularly in conjunction with exophthalmos) suggests hyperthyroidism, while swelling in the parotid area may mean infectious disease (mumps), duct obstruction or tumor of the gland. Enlarged cervical lymph nodes can result from infection, inflammation, allergy, leukemia, Hodgkin's disease, lues or tuberculosis. Jugular vein distention may indicate right-sided congestive heart failure or obstruction of the vena cava.

Hirsuitism can be a symptom of Cushing's disease or an indication of prolonged corticosteroid therapy. Patchy baldness often accompanies lupus erythematosus or tertiary lues.

The skin can be cyanotic from heart disease; pallid from anemia, hypotension, leukemia or approaching syncope; flushed from fever, apprehension, alcoholism, hypertension, belladonna drug ingestion, hyperthyroidism or polycythemia; yellow from liver disease; purplish-brown from porphyrism or bronzed from Gaucher's disease or hemolytic anemia. Numerous punctate petechial hemorrhages of the face, neck and forearms suggest idiopathic thrombocytopenic purpura, leukemia, blood dyscrasias or clotting defects. Striae about the neck with numerous purple capillary branches occur with advanced cirrhosis.

The hands may tremble from hyperthyroidism, apprehension, paralysis agitans, senility, multiple sclerosis or epilepsy. Clubbing of the terminal phalanges of the fingers occurs with poor oxygenation of cardiac interseptal defects or any cardiac or pulmonary disease of long standing. The nail beds are excellent sites for the detection of cyanosis. The hands may feel warm with thyrotoxicosis or infections.

Hyperfunction of the anterior pituitary lobe can result in gigantism if it occurs during body development or acromegaly if it develops after puberty. Dwarfism can be a result of pituitary hypofunction, rickets, achondroplasia or osteogenesis imperfecta. Bowed legs and poor gait can be caused by early rickets. Swollen ankles may signify kidney disease or right-sided heart failure. Barrel chest with dyspnea may occur with emphysema or chronic air passage obstruction.

REVIEWING THE QUESTIONNAIRE

Any questionnaire is only as good as the information derived from its use. Patients are sometimes reticent about confiding certain facts to a dentist whom they erroneously think is concerned only with oral health. The concept of treating a total patient is foreign to them, and they are unaware that systemic conditions may require alteration of our treatment plan or anesthetic procedures. Other patients will not supply information about certain conditions because they are genuinely unaware of their existence or because they are embarrassed by them.

The questionnaire is intentionally repetitive in certain aspects so as to approach a disease state from different directions in an attempt to overcome subterfuge or ignorance. For the patient who is aware of his present status and past history, recognition of names in a listing of specific disease states can provide a means of directing the interview without the need for circuitous questioning.

From other patients, pertinent information must be elicited where we can find it. Certainly, one who is under the care of a physician, who takes medication regularly, or who has been hospitalized within the past two years, is to be suspected of some illness. Persistence in questioning about these points will often bring to light some facts which the patient would not, otherwise, have volunteered. The identity of the attending physician should be ascertained in order to facilitate consultation should it prove desirable. A careful pharmacological history is essential, care being taken to note not only which drugs are involved but also the disease(s) being treated. If the patient does not know the names of drugs he takes, check with his physician. If you are unfamiliar with a drug, look it up in a suitable reference source such as the *Physician's Desk Reference to Pharmaceutical Specialties and Biologicals** (a copy of which should be in every office).

Habitual use of tranquilizers or sedatives may indicate a particularly

* Medical Economics, Inc., Oradell, N. J., Litton Publications, 1971.

unstable personality and suggest the possibility of tolerance to sedative drugs we may administer, thereby necessitating the increase of the dosage or the elimination of certain agents. There is cross-tolerance between many sedative drugs. Patients taking stimulants too soon before treatment may require greater amounts of sedative drugs. Beware of the patient who medicates himself for colds or other conditions without following a rational regimen and the person who takes drugs, such as reducing pills, which he does not tell you about because he does not consider them medicine, since (in his estimation) no disease state is involved.

Questioning about allergies should begin with generalities (pollens, foods, drugs) and proceed to specifics about previous reactions of any kind. Presence of some allergic phenomena is a relative indication of the possibility of other allergies.

Persons who smoke excessively usually have decreased vital capacity, resulting from some pulmonary congestion, which can render them poor candidates for agents that depress the respiratory center. Certainly one who admits to heavy smoking and coughs frequently should be suspect (particularly if the cough is productive). Persistent coughing also may be a symptom of underlying cardiac or pulmonary disease.

Drinkers respond poorly to analgesic and hypnotic drugs. There is a definite alcohol-barbiturate cross-tolerance, and chronic alcoholism can lead to impaired liver function which interferes with normal drug detoxification, producing excessive depth and prolonged recovery. Persons taking narcotics similarly exhibit bizarre behavior under anesthesia. Like alcoholics, they tend to prevaricate, miss appointments and be financially irresponsible.

Abnormal thirst and excessively frequent voiding, possibly coupled with recent weight loss, suggest the presence of diabetes. Pains in the chest or inability to perform normal activities suggest coronary pathology, and a requirement for more than one pillow at night, shortness of breath or ankle edema during the day may indicate congestive heart failure. Marked changes in equilibrium, vision, hearing or taste may suggest central nervous system lesions. Persistent headaches may mean hypertension or central nervous system lesions.

Patients with a heart murmur may have a history of rheumatic fever requiring prophylactic measures. Damaged heart valves usually render the patient especially vulnerable to hypoxia. Fainting may mean hypotension or emotional instability. Patients with asthma, prostatitis or glaucoma should not be given belladonna drugs. Asthmatics or bronchitics may not tolerate any respiratory depression and anemics can be quite intolerant of hypoxia. Pregnant women should probably be spared any relatively deep sedation and, for all women, procedures are best not scheduled during their menstrual periods. A history of hepatitis, mononucleosis or tuberculosis may necessitate special precautions against contagion.

Every bit of information can be valid. Bachelors, widows and widowers tend to be poorly or marginally nourished. The nature of a patient's occupation may suggest adequate recovery from previous illnesses or may, if a change of occupation was necessitated for medical reasons, signify a relatively poor risk status. Familial history (blood relations) of diabetes, heart disease or cancer may suggest a special susceptibility to these diseases. Previous bad anesthetic experience may suggest drug intolerance, allergy or idiosyncrasy.

SPECIFIC CONDITIONS

Heart Disease

A situation whereby there is impairment of the functional capacity of the heart is termed *cardiac decompensation*. The basic symptoms, which develop gradually, are shortness of breath on mild exertion, pitting edema of the ankles, increase in weight and prominently distended neck veins.

As the pumping efficiency of the heart diminishes, the pressure head propelling the blood declines, fluid accumulates in the body and venous pressure increases. The name, *congestive heart failure*, refers to the condition of stasis that ensues. Respiratory capacity is diminished as fluid accumulates in the lungs (left heart failure) and interferes with gaseous exchange so that increased demands concomitant with physical activity cannot be met, and dyspnea, or shortness of breath, results. Since the lungs fill when the patient is lying flat, and he cannot breathe in this position, he adopts the practice of sleeping on several pillows in order to promote collection of the edema fluid in the lung bases and to maintain ventilatory capacity at a sufficient level. If despite this practice he may still be awakened during the night by shortness of breath, the condition is severe indeed.

Fluid increases in the body as the blood flows sluggishly. Body weight tends to increase, the abdomen enlarges and dependent areas (ankles and legs) swell as the day progresses, but reapproach normal with bed rest. Retention of blood in the vessels raises the blood pressure and causes venous distention, particularly observable in the jugular veins. The rapidity of weight gain provides some indication of the acuteness with which the failure is developing. These patients are often taking diuretics, and when they give a history of such medication in the presence of other symptoms, congestive failure with some degree of decompensation must be considered.

The risk for dental treatment and for sedation depends on the degree of failure. With only mild decompensation, treatment can be performed and will be facilitated by premedication with barbiturates, but in more severe cases only emergency procedures should be attempted. Nitrous oxide analgesia is particularly beneficial, since there is no direct myocardial depression as there may be with barbiturates or other drugs. However, proper management and effective sedation are more important than choice of agent for mild sedation.

Patients suffering from *coronary artery disease* often present a greater risk than those with heart failure. Attacks are more sudden and overwhelming and carry the potential of becoming irreversible and proceeding to coronary occlusion and death. The major symptoms are severe substernal pain often radiating to the left shoulder and arm *(angina pectoris)* and severe shortness of breath. The pain tends to be precipitated by exertion or excitement and relieved by rest and vasodilator drugs. Long-term management for these patients usually includes use of nitroglycerin, which dilates the coronary vessels, to relieve attacks.

Dental treatment planning depends on the frequency and severity of attacks. These patients do not tolerate emotional stress well and some routine sedation is beneficial. The nitroglycerin tablets may be taken prophylactically and should be immediately available at all times during treatment to be taken if the need arises. More rapid relief, if urgently necessary, can be obtained by having the patient inhale amyl nitrite. If the attacks are severe and almost daily in frequency, only emergency treatment should be attempted.

Patients with a history of *coronary occlusion (coronary thrombosis, myocardial infarction)* should be spared elective procedures for at least six months following an attack until some healing of the lesion has occurred and some stability has been restored to heart action. The usual history is one of hospitalization followed by a period of convalescence at home. The symptoms include dyspnea and angina-like pains not relieved by nitrites or rest.

Treatment, with careful local anesthetic technique, mild sedation to allay apprehension and lessen excitement, and short appointments, follows basically the same precautions as for angina. These patients are often taking anticoagulants (dicumarol, coumadin, heparin) and the dosage should be adjusted, upon consultation with the attending physician, while local measures are applied for control of hemorrhage.

Hypertension, like angina, is a symptom of underlying disease rather than a disease entity in itself. This is not to be confused with the mild, transitory elevations of systolic pressure experienced by normal persons as a result of exercise or emotional stress. Chronic hypertension is often accompanied by kidney or brain damage and cardiac changes.

Sedation to allay apprehension is beneficial, and effective local anesthesia is mandatory. The New York Heart Association is on record as favoring the use of epinephrine in local anesthetic solutions to enhance anesthesia if no more than 10 ml. of a 1:50,000 solution is injected, slowly and extravascularly, at each visit. The patient should be allowed to rest postoperatively, all anesthetic injections should be made only after negative aspiration, and it is best that sedation is mild.

Possibly as many as one-fifth of chronic hypertensive patients eventually develop cerebral symptoms and stroke. Any history of previous stroke (cerebrovascular accident [CVA], cerebral apoplexy, cerebral hemorrhage, cerebral thrombosis), frequent syncope, speech defects, paresthesia or paralysis of an extremity are significant. The symptoms of an episode can include intense headache, vomiting, drowsiness, convulsions and paralysis.

Appointments should be short. Sedation is helpful but should be administered carefully because, if carried to the point of extreme drowsiness or depression, it can depress cerebral circulation and possibly precipitate cerebral thrombosis. Elective treatment should be deferred for at least six months after a stroke.

Valvular heart disease, causing insufficiency or stenosis of one or more valves, may interfere with normal flow in the heart or permit regurgitation of blood. Possible causes of this scarring of the heart valves include rheumatic fever, inflammatory rheumatism, lupus erythematosus, chorea, periarteritis nodosa and St. Vitus' dance. After the acute disease has subsided, permanent heart damage in the form of scarred valves may persist throughout life and make itself evident in the form of a murmur. Loudness of the murmur, however, does not indicate the amount of damage present which should be evaluated on the basis of functional capacity. Presence of murmur should not be used as the sole diagnostic criterion since it may not be heard in some patients with scarred valves and may occasionally be heard (systolic murmur) in young, healthy persons.

Valvular involvement does not, in itself, contraindicate sedation if the patient is reasonably able to carry on normal activity. However, it should be remembered that there is impaired efficiency of the heart which may have led to decompensation. At all times, these patients tend to be less tolerant of hypoxia than the average person, but with properly managed sedation, hypoxia should not occur. Finally, patients with rheumatism may be receiving corticosteroids whose dosage may have to be adjusted or reinstituted (in the case of recent cessation), since the adrenal cortex may be depressed and lack of autogenous steroids can predispose to a hypotensive episode under sedation.

Congenital heart disease, similarly, does not contraindicate the use of sedative methods if the patient has functional capacity within the normal limits. Degree of decompensation can be gauged on the basis of information volunteered by the patient as to exertional capacity and from observation of cyanosis, clubbing of fingers and evidence of retardation of growth and maturity.

Since there is bound to be some impairment of cardiac function, sedation should be maintained at light levels and patients should be well oxygenated throughout. Prophylactic antibiotics are recommended as with a history of rheumatic heart disease.

Ventilatory Impairment

Dyspnea, or difficult respiration, may be seen in the elderly and obese, persons in poor physical condition, and in persons with a history of emphysema, angina pectoris, coronary insufficiency, asthma, bronchitis, pneumonia or arteriosclerosis. In general, older people breathe more slowly than the young, and respiratory rate accelerates with exertion and emotion. Harsh breathing may result from foreign bodies in the air passages, edema of the glottis, hypertrophied tonsils and adenoids, nasal obstructions and neoplastic or infectious swellings in, or encroaching upon, the airway.

Bronchitis, or inflammation of the tracheobronchial tree, can be acute with eventual healing and return to normal or chronic with fibrotic and atrophic changes in the bronchial structure. While potentially dangerous in debilitated patients and those with chronic pulmonary or cardiac disease, acute bronchitis is usually mild, often developing from an acute upper respiratory infection. Symptoms include those of an acute upper respiratory infection with general malaise, low-grade fever and sore throat, plus pains in the back and a cough which is dry at first but, after a few days, produces a mucopurulent secretion. Fever lasts a few days but the cough may persist for weeks.

Chronic bronchitis may continue for years (with chronic cough) leading to lessened chest expansion and vital capacity. Accumulation of exudate from the infected mucosa, with loss of pulmonary elasticity, predisposes to respiratory obstruction.

Sedation should not be attempted until an acute episode has passed and an adequate convalescent period has elapsed. Deep sedation (particularly by barbiturates which sensitize laryngeal reflexes) should be avoided because of extra susceptibility to coughing spasms, laryngospasm or bronchospasm and because the barbiturates, being parasympathomimetic, may increase the amount of secretions. Nitrous oxide does not irritate the tracheobronchial tree, hence does not stimulate secretions.

Bronchiectasis, often secondary to bronchial obstruction or infection, is a chronic infectious disease producing dilation and thickening of the terminal bronchi and is most common in the lower lobes of the lungs. Symptoms include cough (either dry or with a purulent exudate), occasional hemoptysis, exertional dyspnea and recurrent acute respiratory infections. Fever, malaise, loss of weight, fetid breath and pallor may be accompanied by clubbing of the fingers as impaired lung drainage interferes with ventilation. Vital capacity is diminished and the large amount of mucopurulent secretions in the tracheobronchial tree represents a definite anesthetic risk; a partial obstruction may become total.

Emphysema is a state of distention and inelasticity of the lung alveoli or smaller bronchioles leading to an effective reduction in the functioning area of alveolar membrane available for gaseous exchange. The lungs slowly increase in size, the thoracic cage tends to assume the inspiratory position, and the diaphragm becomes low and flat. Lessening of the normally negative intrapleural pressure requires increased inspiratory effort. Vital capacity and tidal volume diminish while residual volume (air remaining in the lungs after extreme expiratory effort) increases. Hypoxia and elevated carbon dioxide levels follow from loss of gas exchange capability. Pulmonary arterial hypertension and right ventricular hypertrophy with congestive heart failure are important complications.

Patients exhibit wheezing, tiring chronic cough, dyspnea and hyperinflated chest sometimes fixed in the inspiratory position (barrel chest). The course of the disease is one of slow, gradually progressing deterioration leading to disability. Pharmacological depression of respiratory activity (as is possible with deep sedation) must be scrupulously avoided, but mild sedation to avoid the increased metabolic oxygen demands of excitement or apprehension may be beneficial. Nitrous oxide analgesia, which does not depress respiration, may be indicated if respiratory function is adequate for inhalation of sufficient gas. Since the system becomes acclimated to a high carbon dioxide level, too vigorous oxygenation may deprive the respiratory center of sufficient stimulus.

Asthma, a condition with recurrent paroxysms of a characteristically wheezing type of dyspnea, due to a narrowing of the lumens of the bronchi and bronchioles, is usually associated with an inherited allergic constitution. Precipitating allergens can include pollens, molds, animal dander or, less frequently, foods or drugs. The frequency and severity of attacks may be influenced by humidity, temperature change, fatigue, endocrine changes (menstruation, pregnancy, menopause, puberty) and emotional stress.

The symptoms of an attack include a sense of tightness in the chest, dyspnea, wheezing and cough. Acute episodes often end with pronounced coughing and expectoration of a thick bolus of sputum clearing the airway and bringing a sensation of relief. Respiration is often normal between attacks.

No treatment should be attempted during an acute attack. At other times mild sedation, avoiding respiratory depression, is useful for diminishing the emotional stress that can bring on an attack. Patients must be well oxygenated at all times and irritating gases should be avoided. (Nitrous oxide is nonirritating.)

Pulmonary edema is a condition of excess fluid in the alveolar sacs or interstitial lung tissue. The basic causative mechanisms are increased pulmonary capillary pressure secondary to left heart failure, direct damage to the alveolocapillary membranes or accumulation of intra-alveolar fluid caused by inadequate drainage of the tracheobronchial tree.

Pulmonary edema often follows myocardial infarction but may result from some other cause as well, and serves as a parameter to gauge the extent of cardiac failure. Alveolocapillary damage can be a sequel to pulmonary infection, inhalation of chemical irritants (ammonia, acid fumes, chlorine, corrosive dust), or trauma such as chest injuries or sudden atmospheric decompression (bends). Edema in the tracheobronchial tree can follow depressed states where fluid elimination is inadequate, and these states include drug overdosage and terminal circulatory failure.

Occurrence usually involves discrete attacks but in more severe cases symptoms may be persistent. There may be a cough and a wheezing type of breathing because of bronchiolar spasm. The patient experiences dyspnea, orthopnea and a feeling of chest constriction.

Hypoxia is common and may be a contraindication for sedation. Airway patency will be difficult to maintain under all conditions and impossible if the respiration is depressed. Tracheobronchial irritation predisposes to laryngospasm or bronchospasm. Concomitant cardiac decompensation also militates against sedative management.

Breath holding test. One effective means of estimating the functional reserve of a patient with cardiovascular or pulmonary disease is to observe the results of mild exertion such as climbing a flight of stairs. Since this is not practical in most dental offices, a convenient substitute would be to ascertain how long such an individual can hold his breath.

After resting a few minutes, the patient should take a deep breath and hold it as long as possible while pinching his nostrils closed. A normal individual should reach 35 to 45 seconds with little difficulty. Duration of breath holding for less than 15 seconds should be viewed with suspicion especially if there is other evidence of cardiovascular or respiratory disease.

Metabolic Diseases

Diabetes Mellitus

Development of diabetes, a disorder of carbohydrate metabolism due to insufficient production of insulin by the pancreas, is often thought to be strongly influenced by hereditary factors determined by careful recording of familial history. The primary metabolic defect involves decreased ability to properly utilize carbohydrates for production of energy. Blood glucose becomes elevated and may reach the point where it exceeds the renal threshold and spills over into the urine (glycosuria). Incomplete combustion of fats causes accumulation of toxic ketone bodies, such as acetone, in the body. Acetone, like sugar, appears in elevated quantities in the blood and urine and may also be detectable in the breath.

Onset tends to be sudden in the young but gradual and insidious in older persons whose diabetes is often detected only on routine urine examination. The most common symptoms are excessive urine output, thirst, hunger, weight loss, weakness, itching and dry skin. Blood and urine can be shown by test to have elevated sugar levels.

Daily maintenance of therapy is managed by the patient himself so that diabetics, by virtue of their own regular urine testing, tend to be particularly well informed of their current status. Mild cases often can be managed by diet control alone. Moderate diabetics may respond to the oral insulin substitutes (Diabinese, Orinase, Dymelor).

Patients with well-controlled diabetes experience few complications and are able to carry on relatively normal activities. However, all diabetics tend to heal slowly and to develop premature arteriosclerosis and coronary disease. If there is doubt about the degree of control, question the patient about abnormal thirst, weight loss or urinary output.

Never sedate an uncontrolled diabetic, since he is a poor candidate for withstanding stress, and emotional stress increases glycemia. Always consider the special insulin requirements of a patient with an empty stomach prior to sedation and decrease or skip the morning dose after consultation with the attending physician. Schedule the case early in the day so that fasting is not unnecessarily prolonged even though there is little chance of harm resulting from moderately altered blood sugar level for only a short period. If any insulin is taken and the patient does not eat, keep a source of sugar handy. If only very mild sedation (such as nitrous oxide analgesia) is contemplated, allow the patient a light meal. Cancel the procedure if the patient does not feel well.

Thyroid Function

The thyroid gland produces hormones that influence growth and metabolism. Basically, the disease entities associated with thyroid pathology result from the effects of excessive or insufficient production of hormone.

Hyperthyrodism (thyrotoxicosis, exophthalmic goiter) is characterized by nervousness, weakness, sensitivity to heat, sweating, hyperactivity, weight loss despite increased appetite, tremor and palpitation. There is often a swelling anteriorly in the neck at the site of the gland and exophthalmos (protruding eyeballs), which imparts a frightened, staring appearance. Technically, exophthalmos exists when the white of the eye is visible for 360 degrees around the pupil even when it is at rest. This is of itself not pathognomonic of hyperthyroidism, but with its presence the disease should be suspected.

In hyperthyroidism the heart is overactive (often enlarged) and there is a tendency toward tachycardia, atrial fibrillation, increased pulse pressure and headache. There is often tremor of the extremities and patients may report diarrhea, vomiting, nausea, abdominal pains and polyuria. These patients usually exhibit nervous manifestations, and these together with the commonly seen tolerance to sedative drugs, create a requirement for unusually large doses to achieve effective sedation. With the overactivity of the heart, cardiac disease is frequent. Treatment should be postponed, if possible, until the condition is controlled. At all times the elevated metabolic rate increases the oxygen requirement. Increased sensitivity to epinephrine necessitates careful and slow local anesthetic injection.

Hypothyroidism (myxedema) shows many symptoms that are the opposite of those seen for oversecretion of hormone. These patients tend to be sluggish, underactive, sleepy and constipated. They often feel chilly, exhibit cold, dry skin and gain weight easily. Bradycardia, low pulse pressure and lowered cardiac tonus lead to decreased cardiac output, cardiac failure and edema. In children, underactive thyroid function can cause cretinism with subnormal mental and physical development (especially secondary sexual characteristics), thick, dry skin, sparse, thick hair and delayed dentition.

These patients are particularly intolerant of sedative drugs; they tend to show an exaggerated response to only small doses and to recover full consciousness quite slowly. Any cardiac hypofunction should be managed symptomatically.

Adrenal Insufficiency

Adrenal cortical hypofunction, characterized by weakness, abnormal pigmentation of the skin and mucous membranes, weight loss, hypotension, hypoglycemia and gastrointestinal symptoms, is often of a chronically insidious and progressive nature (*Addison's disease*). Such patients withstand stress poorly and are candidates for hypotensive crises or shock from relatively minor stress or mild sedative depression. Prolonged therapy with adrenocorticosteroids (cortisone, hydrocortisone), for whatever reason, depresses the secretive capability of the adrenal cortex with a similar result. Assume that there may be adrenal insufficiency if the patient has regularly taken adrenocorticosteroids within the past six months. Adrenal cortical atrophy is often accompanied by a degeneration of the thyroid gland.

Upon consultation with the attending physician, recently interrupted steroid therapy may be resumed a few days prior to treatment. Pathologically depressed adrenal cortical activity should be carefully evaluated before sedation is attempted. With proper management these patients usually can be expected to react in a normal fashion.

Liver Disease

Liver disease, possibly interfering with carbohydrate or protein metabolism, prothrombin formation or drug detoxification, should be suspected if there is a yellowish jaundice of the skin, sclerae or conjunctivae. Infectious hepatitis is more common in the young and occurs more often in the late autumn; it is characterized by fever, malaise, loss of apetite, lymphadenopathy and an enlarged tender liver. Recent blood administration, parenteral injection or exposure to others with jaundice may furnish a significant clue. Some of the currently used drugs can produce jaundice (chlorpromazine, methyltestosterone and oral contraceptives) as an allergic response. Actual jaundice may be preceded several days before by dark urine.

Cirrhosis associated with chronic alcohol ingestion and malnourishment results in impaired hepatic function and retarded drug detoxification. Recovery from sedative agents (particularly the faster acting barbiturates) is prolonged and excessive depression results as dosage accumulates.

It is incumbent upon the practitioner to take extra steps to protect himself, his staff and his other patients from contagion from patients with a recent history of infectious hepatitis. Disposable hypodermic supplies should be used in all patients but are mandatory in those who have had infectious hepatitis in the previous three years. Scratches or cuts on the operator's hands should be protected by rubber gloves.

Weight Changes

Weight changes can be as significant as static conditions of overweight or underweight. While obesity may be just the result of overeating, it may also reflect abnormal thyroid, pituitary or gonadal function or the retention of fluid of renal or cardiac disease.

Slow weight loss occurs with many chronic illnesses. Rapid weight loss may warn of malignancy, hormonal (hyperthyroid) or metabolic (diabetes) dysfunction or the nutritional deficiency and drug therapy frequently associated with dieting. The amphetamines so commonly included in diet pills, are mono-amine oxidase inhibitors which can lead to hypotensive episodes if a blood level exists when narcotics are administered. It seems, too, that local anesthetics lack their usual reliable potency in patients on amphetamines.

Female Conditions

Most women experience some heightened irritability during and immediately prior to their menstrual periods.

In the absence of other contraindicating factors, sedation will facilitate dental care by counteracting nervousness or anxiety.

Nitrous oxide analgesia may be safely used for pregnant women but most other sedative management is relatively contraindicated (especially in the first trimester and the last month or so). Most sedative drugs pass the placenta and, while the mother may do well, the fetus can possibly be depressed to an excessive degree. Nitrous oxide, it seems, does not depress the fetus and, if properly maintained, analgesia presents no hypoxic hazard. The duration of analgesia maintenance should be as short as is consistent with operative requirements, and the lowest possible concentration of nitrous oxide should be used. The attending obstetrician should be consulted and, for medicolegal reasons, if he flatly refuses permission and will not be dissuaded from this view, it is preferable to forgo use of analgesia and defer any treatment of an elective nature.

Women going through menopause tend to exhibit symptoms which may include nervousness, excitability, hot flashes and chills, lack of vigor, muscle and joint pains, gastrointestinal disturbances, depression, insomnia, palpitation and headache. They respond poorly to the stresses of dental treatment and tend to overreact to pain, anticipated or actual. Their altered mental attitudes may militate against a nasal mask on the face, and for these women premedication can be especially beneficial. It is important, however, to ascertain that the symptoms are truly those of the hormonal imbalances of menopause rather than those of coexisting organic disease.

FUNCTIONAL RESERVE CLASSIFICATION

A determination should be made not only of the patient's ability to engage in normal daily activities but also of his cardiovascular reserves for meeting the increased demands of stress. One who exhibits no dyspnea upon normal exertion usually presents no special risk. With mild dyspnea from such exertion as climbing a flight of stairs, the risk status can still be good if all other points are negative. As exertional capacity diminishes, the indication for medical consultation increases. Mild sedation, with good local anesthesia, is of value in reducing emotional stresses for these patients, but their limits of tolerance must be defined and never exceeded. Patients with constant dyspnea and orthopnea (who may have to rest numerous times when climbing a flight of stairs if they are able to negotiate them at all) at all times present a serious risk for sedation or for dental treatment performed in any manner. Not only should sedative depression be avoided but also all except emergency dental treatment.

The ultimate responsibility rests with the dentist, who should make his determination to proceed, and how to proceed, only after thoroughly exploring all investigative avenues.

5 | Monitoring

The potency of today's general anesthetic and sedative agents necessitates accurate observation of the patient's reactions in order to avoid administration of an overdose and to provide for safe maintenance. Ideally, the optimal dose is that which provides suitable conditions for the operative procedure yet involves the use of the least amount of agent(s) and deranges the least physiology.

There are no ironclad rules for determination of dosage, since effects vary from patient to patient and from one administration to another for the same individual. It is essential, therefore, that there be a means of gauging the depth of depression for any given patient at any given moment.

STAGES OF ANESTHESIA

The grouping of anesthetic occurrences into stages and substages, called planes, was first postulated by Guedel. He cataloged objective symptoms ensuing from the obtundation of certain physiological responses at varying levels of anesthesia. This sequence, divided into four stages, with the third stage in four planes, is used as a signpost for the blocking or modification of various neural (reflex) responses. There are limitations, though, to this system of observation, therefore rendering sole reliance upon it a procedure to be avoided. As a teaching tool it remains of great value. For that reason it is presented here despite our limitation to sedative techniques which produce only first-stage (analgesia) depth.

The signs and stages are best seen with those agents providing a slow induction and a gradual elevation of blood level. Guedel's classification applies essentially to the administration of ether to the unpremedicated patient. For such an anesthesia the signs indicate depth with relative accuracy.

In many modern clinical situations, with the agents presently available, these signs are often obscured or lacking and careful monitoring of the patient's vital signs (pulse, respiration, blood pressure) is employed to determine depth.

In our sedative management we see, basically, one set of signs—those of the first stage (analgesia). We are able to expand this stage greatly and can see much variation in the amount of depression produced without ever leaving it. For our purposes second stage (excitement) symptoms are, by their very presence, indication that we have exceeded our limits and are beginning to produce general anesthesia. It is possible, with a dose just the least bit subhypnotic, to bring a patient to the excitement stage and to maintain him there without ever carrying him deeper. This is potentially dangerous to the patient and does not allow us to perform any treatment. It is to be strenuously avoided.

The signs and stages of Guedel, studied in the proper context, do provide a guide for the study of anesthetic maintenance and, as such, they are presented here.

STAGE I • ANALGESIA—commences with the beginning of anesthesia and continues to the loss of consciousness. By definition, the patient is under the effects of our agents but remains technically awake.

Respiration is essentially normal. It exhibits its normal rhythmic pattern including a shorter, active inspiratory phase and a longer, passive expiratory phase. Inspiration results from active muscular effort and expiration represents a return to the resting state through intrinsic elastic recoil of the involved muscles. Muscular tone remains normal elsewhere in the body.

The eyes exhibit normal voluntary movement. Eyelid and lash reflexes are unchanged and the pupil reacts to light.

Protective pharyngeal and laryngeal reflexes are present. Foreign matter falling back into the throat can be coughed up as in the totally awake individual; but the patient will be less aware of its presence and will tolerate these particles more. While he can expectorate and bring up these offending particles, he is less likely to be stimulated to do so.

Patients in Stage I do, in fact, tolerate almost everything more, including pain. They perceive pain sensation but are less likely to object to it. There is a euphoria that makes everything seem a little less offensive. It becomes easier to maintain a wide-open mouth for long periods of time, to remain quiet without movement of the trunk or limbs, to refrain from rinsing or spitting out, and so on. The patient floats along with us and yet alone in his own world of reverie.

Amnesia is often present but this is one of the most variable facets of analgesia maintenance. A very common occurrence, though, is an altered perception of the passage of time (a form of amnesia). Patients just do not know how long they were under. Perhaps this is one reason why they do not mind prolonged procedures—they do not perceive them as being so long.

In lighter phases of analgesia patients are more subject to positive suggestion. Induction techniques borrowed from the hypnotist can potentiate our agents and are of great value. As patients reach deeper levels in Stage I they lose their suggestibility as they lose further contact with their surroundings.

They can communicate and when they do they may describe a condition of comfort, warmth, light-headedness, dizziness, lethargy and euphoria. They often feel their limbs to be very heavy. Of course, not every patient feels every symptom every time.

Stage I has some breadth as do all the stages. Patients may be light or deep in Stage I and exhibit different signs. Deep Stage I begins to resemble light Stage II. The boundaries between the stages exist only in books, not in patients. In practice the transition from one stage to another is not seen in any definite manner. A patient deep in Stage I, while still maintaining some consciousness and reaction to external stimuli, may begin to exhibit the irregularity of respiration that is the classic sign of Stage II. This irregularity will not, however, be nearly as marked as it will be later when Stage II is truly reached.

Maintenance in Stage I, coordinated with local anesthesia when necessary, facilitates virtually all areas of dental treatment and may be continued for long periods of time. The symptoms of obtundation of memory, perception of time and space and integrative functions, are evidence of depression of the higher centers, those most recently evolved phylogenetically.

Remember, the stage of analgesia can also serve as the first step in a general anesthetic induction. With modern techniques of intravenous barbiturate general anesthetic induction, it is traversed so rapidly as not to be seen at all. By suitable methods, however, it can be sustained and used as a modality in itself.

STAGE II • EXCITEMENT—commences with the loss of consciousness and continues through a period of irregular respiration until respiratory regularity is reestablished. Respiration is irregular in both rate and depth. The rhythm is disturbed. Expiration can become an active muscular effort, shortening its duration and its relative proportion of the cycle. There can be periods of breath holding of varying duration.

STAGE II • EXCITEMENT
    Respiration—irregular
    Eyeballs—oscillate
    Eyes—react to light
    Pupils—moderately dilated
    Muscles—increased movement and
        tonicity
    Reflexes—some obtunded late in
        stage
    Patient—unconscious
    No treatment possible

The eyeballs oscillate due to imbalance of ocular muscle tone. The various suspensory and controlling muscles inserting into the eyeball receive their motor innervation from different cranial nerves which are anesthetized at differing levels of depth. The result is a loss of the balanced antagonism usually present in the awake person and this leads to the oscillation described.

The pupils, which were normally open in analgesia, tend to dilate moderately but continue to react to light until deep in the stage where such reaction is reduced.

The eyelid reflex is obtunded at the lower limits of the excitement stage.

The most obvious sign is that of muscular tonicity and movement, hence the term excitement. Motor innervation to skeletal muscles is not obtunded but various cortical inhibitory mechanisms are. The result is a random muscular reaction characterized by increased tone and, often, uninhibited movement with flailing of the extremities. The jaws are clenched and the patient moves quite actively and powerfully. Dental treatment, as well as all other procedures, is quite impossible.

The pharyngeal and laryngeal reflexes are obtunded at the lower limits of this stage with the entrance into the stage of surgical anesthesia. It is important to be aware, though, that before these reflexes absent themselves they pass through a time of increased sensitivity. It is deep in the excitement stage that laryngospasm is most likely to occur. One of the reasons, in addition to convenience, that the newer, more rapid induction techniques are employed for general anesthesia is the shortness or absence of excitement stage with the greater degree of safety derived therefrom.

Another of the bad features of Stage II is the greatly increased tendency for vomiting. This results from relative lack of inhibition of the vomiting center.

In sedative management this stage should never be reached. If premonitory signs are present, the level should be lightened.

In general anesthetic inductions this stage is best traversed as rapidly as possible, for no treatment can be performed. Inhibitory checks are absent while reflexes are still active. Higher cerebral centers are depressed with loss of inhibition of secondary centers. This is one of the danger periods of anesthesia during which vomiting and laryngospasm are more common and physical injury may take place. In general anesthesia careful attention should be paid to adequate premedication, proper restraint of the extremities and minimal external sensory stimuli in order to achieve a smooth, rapid passage.

STAGE III • SURGICAL ANESTHESIA—lasts from the onset of automatic, regular respiration to the cessation of spontaneous respiration resulting from central respiratory paralysis due to the action of the anesthetic agent. This stage has been divided into four planes but for our purposes it can be considered as a whole.

STAGE III • SURGICAL ANESTHESIA
Respiration—automatic, regular early in stage, depressed late in stage
Eyeballs—fixed
Eyes do not react to light
Pupils—progressively dilate
Muscle tone decreases
Protective reflexes obtunded

Respiration, as stated previously, is regular at the beginning. As deeper levels are reached, intercostal muscle activity becomes decreased and gradually ceases. Diaphragmatic activity becomes relatively more apparent. Abdominal breathing becomes more pronounced as thoracic breathing lessens. Respiratory exchange becomes progressively reduced until breathing stops at the lower limits of the stage.

The eyeballs become fixed early and the pupils, which were quite constricted at the onset of Stage III, become markedly dilated by the end. Muscle tone decreases gradually until flaccidity is reached near its end.

Most of the reflexes we have been referring to disappear in plane one, but some persist into the second plane. After that point they remain absent. Laryngospasm cannot occur once the laryngeal reflex is obtunded, but aspiration is a real danger. Vomiting can no longer occur and aspiration, if it does occur, most likely involves the debris of our dental treatment (tooth fragments, amalgam crumbs, wedges, and so on). For this reason, endotracheal intubation is especially beneficial for dental treatment performed under general anesthesia. However, for any procedure it is a valuable adjunct for anesthetics maintained at this depth. Intubation is a procedure of sufficient complexity to preclude learning it from a text. Proficiency with this technique can come only from supervised administration of many anesthetics. This is one reason why this text is intended only for teaching sedation techniques and not for general anesthesia. The chapter on general anesthesia (Chap. 17) is intended for background only and not for implementation.

STAGE IV • MEDULLARY PARALYSIS—commences with the cessation of respiration and continues until the failure of circulation. This stage is of academic interest only because it should never be reached, much less maintained. Circulatory collapse (cardiac arrest) should be anticipated before it occurs and immediate steps should be taken to lighten the anesthetic level.

STAGE IV • MEDULLARY PARALYSIS
Respiration ceases
Circulatory collapse
Pupils totally dilated
Muscular relaxation is total

Respiratory cessation can be treated by artificial ventilation of the patient with no resulting permanent disability. It is often produced intentionally, in a controlled manner, in the course of anesthetic management. Brain damage occurs only after total lack of cerebral oxygenation for approximately 4 minutes. Artificial oxygenation can be as effective as, or even more effective than, spontaneous ventilation and can definitely prevent brain damage.

Circulatory failure is in a different class entirely. Even the best hospital cardiac arrest teams have only fair records of success. Then too, cardiac arrest is accompanied first by respiratory arrest, and so there are two problems to treat instead of one.

The pupils are totally dilated. The iris appears as large as the pupil. If you happen upon an accident victim and wish to render first-aid treatment, check his pupils. If the victim does not appear to be breathing, seems to have no peripheral pulse and has paralytically dilated pupils, you are dealing with a level of depression equivalent to Stage IV. The prognosis is virtually hopeless, especially with the means for treatment available at roadside. This is why doctors examine the eyes of unconscious patients.

Vital Signs

The signs of anesthesia result from depression of specific areas of functional activity of the brain by the anesthetic agents. Depression of the higher centers of the cortex produces amnesia, stupor and anesthetic sleep. Loss of ability to react to external stimuli signifies depression of the areas of motor coordination. Medullary depression causes failure of the respiratory vasomotor and cardiac centers.

It must always be remembered that the anesthetized patient is not one organ system but an entity. If there is uncertainty as to the depth, always consider the level too deep and lighten the

anesthesia. Intravenously or intramuscularly administered agents cannot be regulated in this manner. Recovery is too slow with these modalities. However, further increments can be avoided and inhalation administration, if concurrent, can be stopped.

It must be emphasized that any detrimental changes in vital signs (respiration, yulse, blood pressure) necessitate immediate steps to lighten the depth of anesthesia. The degree of change dictates the magnitude of measures to be applied.

Only experience with the various agents and modes of administration will enable the neophyte to gauge accurately the depth of anesthesia. It is absolutely essential to maintain close and continuous vigilance during the management in order to be able to discover even small changes in signs and judge the reason for their occurrence.

We monitor with our senses of touch, sight and hearing. With experience everything we perceive about the patient has relevance. By applying our knowledge and common sense, we can transform our observations into appropriate action for safeguarding the patient and maintaining a smooth and pleasant anesthetic.

Monitoring involves observation of the function of various organ systems. In effect, we are performing a continuing physical examination. For expediency, to prevent excessive preoccupation with this anesthetic responsibility and to avoid undue distraction from our operative procedures, we select certain representative indicators of body function and concentrate our attention on them. These indicators are commonly called the vital signs and include pulse, blood pressure and respiration.

In our preoperative evaluation, we noted the patient's vital signs and took appropriate action if we found any to be outside acceptable limits. Anesthesia for these patients can be performed in a hospital or medical treatment can be instituted, by the proper practitioner, to correct any abnormalities.

At the time of anesthesia we are, then, dealing with a patient exhibiting relatively normal and stable vital signs. Monitoring is intended to detect relative changes from our base line of preoperative findings. It is important to consider not only how much of a change has occurred but what percentage of variation it represents from the pretreatment, or preanesthetic, findings. A 10-beat per minute change in pulse is more significant in an adult with a normal of 65 beats than in a child with a normal of 110. When viewed in conjunction with other vital signs, we can make our decision as to what is the appropriate action to take in a given situation.

VITAL FUNCTIONS

Cardiovascular Function

Pulse

The pulse is used as an indicator of the rate and regularity of cardiac contraction. It is observed by palpating a peripheral artery and several are superficial enough for this purpose. The most commonly used is the radial artery palpable on the ventral surface of the wrist just proximal to the joint. Other arteries that serve well are the superficial temporal felt just anterior to the tragus of the ear and the external maxillary which is best palpated as it crosses the inferior border of the mandible. The pulse in the common carotid artery in the neck is easily palpated as well, but this site should not be used routinely. It is reserved for urgent situations where no pulse is felt elsewhere

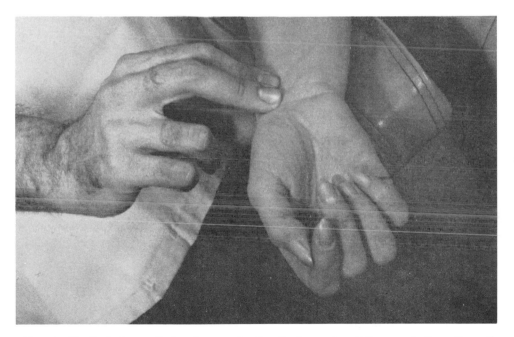

FIG. 4. To feel the radial pulse apply the fleshy pads of fingers (other than the thumb) to the ventral surface of the wrist on the side towards the thumb and just proximal to the wrist joint.

or no blood pressure is found. This site is to be avoided because digital pressure on the carotid sinus located here can cause lowered blood flow to the cerebrum with syncope-like results.

Palpation is performed with the fleshy pad at the tip of any finger other than the thumb, which has its own pulse. Rate is determined by counting beats felt per minute and is expressed in that manner An adequate figure for comparison can be arrived at by counting beats in a 15-second period and multiplying the resultant figure by 4. This is the common method.

Table 1—Average Normal Pulse Rate at Various Ages	
Age	Beats Per Minute
2-5 years	100-130
5-8 years	90-100
8-14 years	80-90
Adult	60-80

Healthy adult males usually have a pulse rate approximating 60 to 80 beats per min.; in females it is often more rapid by as much as 10 beats per min. The normal for children aged 3 to 14 years is 80 to 120 beats per min. and in infants and children younger than 5 it may go as high as 140 to 150 beats per min. for either sex.

Various factors are recognized that modify pulse rate with no pathological significance attached to the differences they cause, especially if on removal there is a return to normal. Warmth speeds the pulse and cold slows it. The rate is faster during exertion and for a short period afterward, as it is also during digestion or a period of mental excitement. Apprehension and fear of anticipated pain in a dental office is a potent pulse rate stimulant. Athletes, characteristically, have slow pulses.

Pulse quality can be as revealing as rate. Within normal limits it should be strong and regular. Weak, thready pulse is related to lowered peripheral blood pressure. Cardiac arrhythmia during anesthesia may be due to hypoxia or carbon dioxide excess and can often be eliminated by oxygenation. Not all arrhythmias are the same. It is important to note the nature of the rhythmic deficit. If an occasional beat is missed, does this happen in a regular sequence (every third beat, every fifth beat) or does it represent a purely random pattern? The more arrhythmic the arrhythmia the more significant it is.

Even the best cardiac rhythm is not perfectly regular. There is often some discernible fluctuation corresponding to respiratory movements. During the inspiratory portion of the respiratory cycle the intrathoracic pressure is diminished, return of blood to the heart is facilitated, and pulse may be accelerated. During expiration, the intrathoracic pressure situation is reversed and pulse rate may be retarded.

Various pressure-sensitive devices, more sensitive than our fingertips, are occasionally substituted for methods of direct palpation. By means of these devices, pulsations may be made to register by such means as a blinking light, a beeping sound, an oscillating needle or a continuous oscilloscope tracing. However, there exists, with this equipment, the possibility of introduction of artifacts caused by extraneous movement or electrical interference, and the possibility of distraction of the operator from the procedures in progress. Definitive interpretation often depends upon a high level of specialized training. The equipment is often delicate, bulky and costly. The fine distinctions obtainable by such means may be highly valuable for major surgical procedures performed with sophisticated anesthetic methods for patients of questionable risk status. But for dental treatment, which involves little physiological alteration with good-risk patients on whom only sedative modalities are used, such equipment is unneccesary. We would do far better to limit ourselves to our own senses for monitoring the more significant of the vital signs in our somewhat gross manner. The information received is more than adequate and we can devote sufficient attention to our operative procedures.

Arterial Blood Pressure

Arterial blood pressure determination is employed as a quantitative means of assessing cardiovascular status. As the heart alternately contracts and relaxes, there occurs a parallel fluctuation of the pressure exerted upon the walls of vessels by the volume of blood contained within them. With ventricular contraction, blood is expelled from the heart into the arterial system more rapidly than it can flow out into tributary vessels or than the vessel walls can stretch to accommodate it. The maximum pressure attained, at the end of the rapid ejection phase, is called the *systolic pressure.* This portion of the cardiac cycle is called systole.

During that portion of the cardiac cycle, called diastole, in which the heart is filling and no further ejection of blood occurs, arterial pressure falls. Immediately prior to the next ventricular contraction, arterial pressure is at its lowest. Blood has flowed out to the peripheral branches of the arterial tree and none has replaced it. The minimal value, the lower limit of blood pressure, is called the *diastolic pressure.* Thus, systolic pressure is an indicator of functional activity (energy output) of the cardiac mechanism and, secondarily, the elasticity or distensibility of the major vessels. Diastolic pressure represents the constant load on the peripheral vessels or, otherwise stated, the resistance the ventricle must overcome

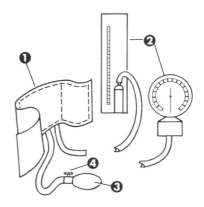

Fig. 5. The parts of a sphygmomanometer include (1) a cuff with an inflatable air bladder, (2) a manometer, either aneroid or mercurial, for measuring the pressure in the system, (3) a squeeze bulb for inflation, and (4) a valve for controlled slow release of pressure. (Courtesy of W. A. Baum and Co., Copiague, New York)

in expelling the volume of blood contained therein. The pulse pressure is the arithmetical difference between systolic and diastolic pressures. Its value will vary with the volume of blood expelled from the heart and with the arterial system's ability to accept it.

Arterial blood pressure is measured, in clinical situations, by a device called a sphygmomanometer. This consists of a cuff wrapped around the upper arm equipped with a means of squeezing the enclosed artery until flow through it is stopped. A recording mechanism indicates the amount of pressure required. Blood pressure can be measured in the thigh as well but this site is seldom used, the arm being more accessible and more convenient. Hemodynamic events within the compressed artery are monitored with a stethoscope. The Bowles type of stethoscope with its flat broad bell and diaphragm is preferred to the Ford with its higher, roughly conical, open-ended type. The

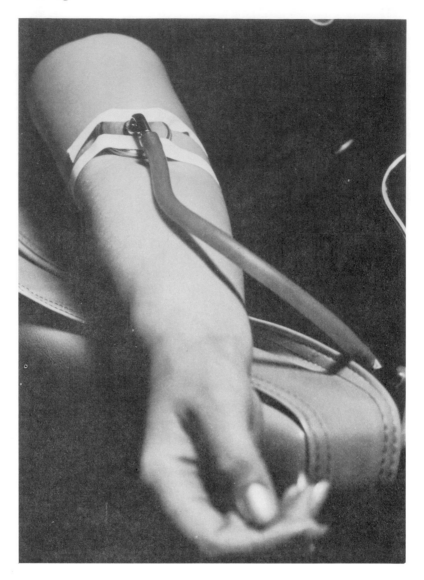

FIG. 6. To use a Bowles type of stethoscope, tape it in place
over the brachial artery just proximal to the elbow joint.

cuff should be of such size as to fit the upper arm without encroaching on the axilla at one side or the antecubital fossa at the other. Properly fitted, it should cover about two-thirds of the upper arm. The stethoscope bell should be so placed as to cover the brachial artery just proximal to the elbow joint. Usually it will be partially covered by the cuff. As in all applications, the diaphragm should be tightly pressed against the skin. A gap between the diaphragm and skin introduces acoustic loss into the stethoscope. The bell can be hand held against the skin or, for prolonged application, can be taped down securely. A stethoscope with a strap to hold the bell in position is available and is commonly used by anesthesiologists.

The varying lengths of upper arms in children make size selection of cuff difficult. Varying widths are available but the variability of the ratio between cuff size and arm length is a prime factor in producing a lack of reliability in blood pressure readings in children. Far more valuable for monitoring cardiac function in children up to 8 or 9 years is the information derived from the use of a precordial stethoscope firmly fixed to the anterior chest wall in the area just medial to the left nipple. The greater thickness of the chest wall in adults, masking sound transmission, and the greater reliability of blood pressure readings, are the reasons why the latter method is more commonly used for older patients.

The cuff is made of a nonstretchable material and contains an inflatable air bladder. It is wrapped around the arm in such a manner as to place the inflat-

able bag between the cuff and the skin and directly over the artery to be compressed. By means of a rubber squeeze bulb the bladder is inflated to a pressure in excess of the presumed systolic pressure and then slowly deflated to return to a state of rest. The cuff should be placed around the arm in a passive state and all occlusive pressure should emanate from the air bladder.

Pressures existent in the system are read from a manometer. This may contain a column of mercury or an air pressure gauge. In effect, we are determining how high a column of mercury can be raised by the pressure exerted in the artery by the force of the flowing blood. The column is calibrated in millimeters and is read in this manner. The air pressure, or aneroid, manometers are calibrated so as to give column-

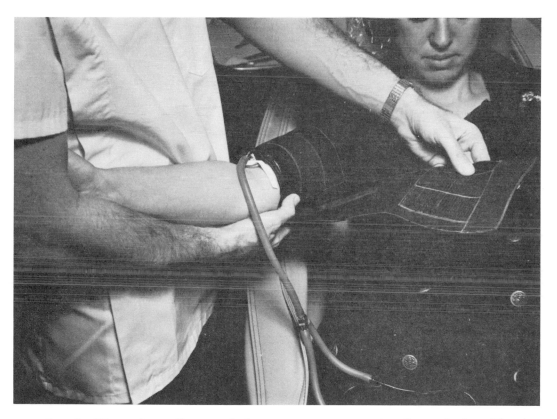

FIG. 7. Wrap the cuff around the upper arm so as to sit passively without occlusive pressure when not inflated.

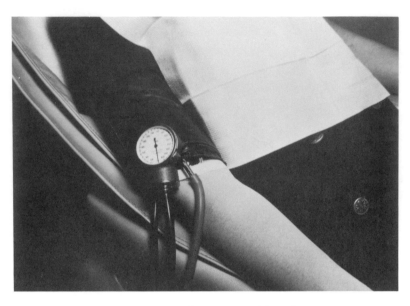

FIG. 8. A stethoscope and an aneroid sphygmomanometer are placed ready for use. The arm is well supported and in a relaxed position.

of-mercury values and are, likewise, calibrated in millimeters.

When blood pressure values are recorded, both systolic and diastolic levels are given. Thus, blood pressure for a healthy young adult may be written as 120/80 and this means systolic pressure of 120 mm. mercury and diastolic pressure of 80 mm. mercury whether taken by mercurial or aneroid sphygomomanometer. We say that blood pressure is 120 over 80. By convention, only even numbers are used.

Blood pressure can be taken by the auscultatory method which involves use of a stethoscope or by the palpatory method which does not. The former technique provides both systolic and diastolic values and is more precise. With the latter method, only systolic level is determined but the procedure is quicker and simpler and usually suffices for moment-to-moment comparisons during a sedative management.

When the auscultatory method is used we listen with a stethoscope placed over the point of maximal pulsation of the brachial artery just proximal to the antecubital fossa. When the artery is not compressed and the lumen is fully open, blood flows through it in laminar fashion and there is no sound. When the cuff is inflated to a pressure higher than the systolic level the artery is occluded; no blood flows through and there is no sound. When the pressure of the air bag on the artery is between that of systolic and diastolic, the artery is compressed but partially open. As blood flows through the compressed segment, turbulence is produced which is transmitted to the vessel walls and surrounding tissues as vibration or sounds which are detectable by stethoscope.

Auscultatory blood pressure determination involves inflation of the cuff to an occluding pressure higher than the presumed systolic pressure and listening with a stethoscope while the bag is

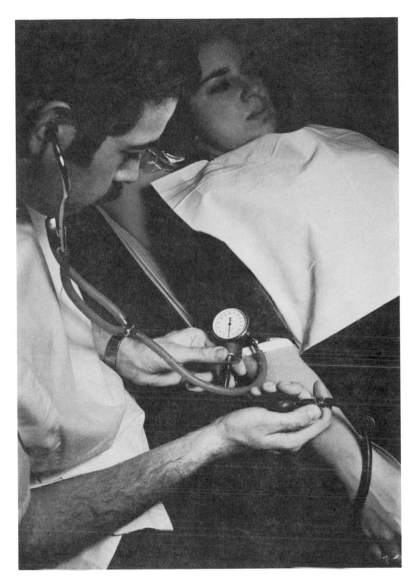

Fig. 9. In palpatory blood pressure determination systolic and diastolic values are read from the manometer dial according to sounds heard during deflation of the cuff.

slowly deflated at the rate of approximately 5 mm. mercury per sec. As inflation pressure falls below the systolic level some blood will spurt through the compressed segment of artery and a sound will be heard. The value registered on the manometer at this point is the systolic pressure. As the inflation pressure continues to decrease, more blood passes through the artery, turbulence is greater and the sounds become louder. When diastolic level is approached, the sound loses its distinct thudlike quality, becomes muffled and then disappears. The point of disappearance is the diastolic level.

During treatment it is not always necessary to obtain such definitive in-

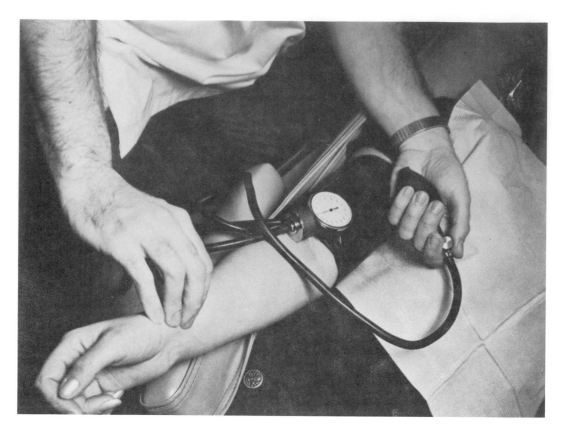

FIG. 10. In palpatory blood pressure determination systolic level is read on the manometer dial as the first radial pulse is felt during slow deflation of the cuff.

formation and a quicker technique, the palpatory method, can be used. Systolic readings tend to be about 4 to 6 mm. lower than those obtained by the auscultatory method and no diastolic level can be estimated. But there is adequate information to gauge momentary fluctuations that might occur.

The cuff is applied in normal fashion and the pulse is palpated at the radial artery of the same arm. No pulse will be felt when the cuff is inflated to a pressure exceeding systolic. The pressure level at which the first pulse is felt at the wrist during deflation of the cuff is the systolic and no further information is obtained.

Releasing inflation pressure too slowly can cause venous stasis distal to the cuff, predisposing to falsely high diastolic and falsely low systolic readings. If the cuff is too wide, readings will be inaccurately low since more of the artery is compressed and some pressure of the blood flow will be dissipated in overcoming resistance. A cuff of insufficient width can give incorrectly high readings.

TABLE 2—AVERAGE NORMAL VALUES FOR ARTERIAL BLOOD PRESSURE AT VARIOUS AGES

In millimeters of Mercury

Age	Systolic	Diastolic
3 years	85-95	45-55
8 years	90-100	50-60
12 years	100-120	60-80
Adult	110-140	70-80

Normal adult male systolic pressure can range from 105 to 150 mm.; in females it is commonly 5 to 10 mm. lower. In children younger than 8 years it is usually in the range of 85 to 100 mm. and at the ages of 8 to 12 years it can be found between 100 and 120 mm. Diastolic pressure can be expected to be between 25 and 50 mm. lower. Pressure often varies upward by 20 to 30 mm. after exertion or during excitement but should soon return to the individual normal after such a period terminates. If the readings are suspect, take several and assume the lowest to be correct. It is not uncommon to see a small drop after the beginning of sedative administration. This often reflects onset of relaxation (loss of anxiety) and can be construed as a return to normal. If there is a further drop, this can signify overdosage. In such a situation, further medication should be avoided until the normal is reestablished. A drop in blood pressure can also be caused by excessive blood loss or surgical manipulation but stimuli of this magnitude are rare in dental treatment. A rise in blood pressure can result from being undersedated or waning of sedative effect, and can be countered by administration of more agent. Too rapid administration of fluids in an intravenous drip infusion can also elevate the blood pressure and, should this occur, the rate should be slowed.

Remember that the sphygmomanometer is a delicate instrument and should be handled with care or it may become inaccurate. Check it occasionally to be certain that the mercury column or gauge needle returns to zero when all cuff pressure is released. If cuff pressure cannot be maintained at a given level, look for an open fitting or a puncture or crack in the tubing or bladder.

Any extraneous movement of the arm or tubing can cause artifacts in the sounds heard during sphygmomanometry. Protect the arm from contact and prevent its movement. Place the tubing in such a manner as to avoid movement, kinks or rubbing.

As a rule it is best not to take blood pressure and administer intravenous fluids in the same arm. If this must be done, always stop the infusion while the cuff is inflated. The cuff acts as a tourniquet and accumulation of fluids can cause the vein to be ruptured.

While care must be exercised in the handling of aneroid sphygmomanometers, it is more urgent with the mercurials. In addition to the other factors, the mercurials have a glass column that can break and a quantity of mercury that can spill. As a rule, they are bulkier than the aneroids which usually have only a small dial that can be clipped directly to the cuff, thereby taking no room and remaining out of the way yet accessible for inspection. Aneroid models are probably better suited for use in a dental treatment room.

Respiratory Function

Proper respiratory function is no less crucial to the well-being of the individual than is correct cardiovascular performance. Optimal tissue oxygenation depends just as much upon pulmonary ventilation as it does upon hemodynamic events. Hence, it behooves us to direct our attention to monitoring of respiratory function throughout the maintenance of the sedated state.

TABLE 3—AVERAGE NORMAL VALUES FOR RESPIRATORY RATE AND TIDAL VOLUME AT VARIOUS AGES		
Age (yrs.)	Rate (per min.)	Tidal Volume (ml)
3	30	100
6	27	150
11	24	200
14	22	250
Adult	16	450-500

We are concerned with the rate, depth and nature of respirations. Information is gained by watching or palpating the chest in its movements. Assuming good mask fit and a properly functioning anesthesia machine, the movements of the breathing bag reflect the nature of respiratory function. In fact, it is sometime advisable to use a nasal mask and administer only oxygen in a case where we do not wish to use nitrous oxide or other inhalation anesthetic, so that the breathing bag will serve as a monitoring device, showing respiratory actions by its movements.

When counting respiratory excursions to determine rate it is necessary to continue for at least 30 sec.—a longer period than that for pulse monitoring. The average adult respiratory rate is about 16 breaths per min. In a 14-year-old it is about 22 per min. and in a 6-year-old approximately 27 per min. Since the rate is slower than that of the pulse, an error of 1 breath per unit of time monitored, multiplied out to a minute, will be proportionately greater in the final determination. This possibly greater source of error is minimized by counting for a longer period and multiplying by a smaller factor in converting to breaths per minute.

The average person is quite capable of exercising voluntary control over respiratory function. A period of breath holding at the beginning of an induction should be recognized as being consciously controlled or influenced and is usually not evidence of a condition requiring remedial action. Breath holding can be the result of reflex action, possibly of vagal origin, but in early induction it is most often voluntary.

There is often marked emotional influence of respiratory function. Fear, apprehension and anxiety often accelerate breathing as they do pulse, and onset of sedation can cause a slowing which is viewed, basically, as a return to the normal rather than as true bradypnea or slowness of respiration.

Bradypnea is, however, to be considered during management as the result of central medullary depression by sedative drugs. The barbiturates, particularly, are potent respiratory depressants. Respiratory depression following administration of narcotics affects depth also but most notably depresses rate. Drugs must be given slowly, in incremental fashion, with attention paid to influence on respiratory function to avoid overdosage. Should drug-induced retardation be seen, no further agent should be given until proper function resumes and the patient should be adequately oxygenated by increasing the percentage of oxygen in the inspired gas mixture, and with manual pressure on the breathing bag if necessary. As a general rule, a respiratory rate in adults, slower than 12 per min., requires corrective action.

The opposite condition tachypnea, or increased respiratory rate, may be so rapid as to interfere with the efficiency of pulmonary ventilation and make it inadequate. Tachypnea can occur without accompanying increase in depth. The age of the patient must be considered, as the rate is normally rapid in children. The degree of rapidity must be considered against the background of departure from individual normal. One of the most common causes of tachypnea is oxygen lack with attendant carbon dioxide excess. Treatment consists of oxygenation by enriching the inspired gas mixture in oxygen content, removal of obstruction, and manual assistance on the breathing bag. Another possible cause is sensation of pain and this should be treated by injection of additional local anesthetic.

Dyspnea, or difficulty in breathing, as opposed to bradypnea, may be caused by mechanical restriction of the intercostal muscles, thoracic cage and diaphragm, or encroachment on the patency of the airway. Mechanical restriction of thoracic movements may be the result of a tight brassiere or corset or pressure on the chest area from objects lying there. The best treatment is prevention. Women should be instructed not to wear corsets or tight girdles, and a tight brassiere can be unfastened without actual removal. Never place any instruments or materials on the patient's chest and always watch the position of your arms and those of your assistants. A fully awake patient can have sufficient reserve to compensate but a sedated one may not.

As relaxation progresses the airway may become compromised. The pharyngeal walls develop a tendency to fall inward and the tongue may fall back. In obese patients this can be particularly marked. Head position should be considered and corrected if necessary. The neck should be fully extended to eliminate kinks in the anatomic airway tube. Pressure behind the gonial angle to protrude the mandible (in a supine patient the pressure should be exerted upward) tends to pull the tongue forward out of the pharynx.

Any accumulated secretions, vomitus or debris should be removed from the oropharynx. Turning the head to the side will facilitate pooling in the cheek rather than in the pharynx. Administration of an antisialagogue such as atropine will minimize the volume of secretions. Remember that even though the patient is still in command of some conscious control, it is diminished and assistance may be required.

Observe the movements of the chest. In an obstructed state the chest will retract as the diaphragm descends in contradistinction to the normal situation in which it should expand. The characteristic rocking motion seen indicates that a free inflow of air is not able to follow the descent of the diaphragm. The movements of the chest are a better indication than those of the bag which may continue even though diminished.

Respiratory activity, which is normally almost soundless, may be accompanied by stertorous or snoring sounds in the presence of partial obstruction. As the loose tissues of the pharyngeal walls, soft palate and tongue fall in, they vibrate with the passage of air. Laryngospasm, either partial or complete, is unlikely in the stage of analgesia produced by sedative agents.

The chest, when it expands, should do so evenly on both sides, signifying expansion of both lungs. This can be seen or palpated. By listening with a stethoscope it is possible to detect sounds of air rushing through the respiratory tubes. Abnormal sounds arising within the air passages or lungs, termed rales, usually mean that there is some fluid contained therein. This is not unusual with a cold or productive cough and is usually heard with pneumonia or emphysema. It is a possible contraindication to general anesthesia but, while worth noting, is less critical with sedative management. When considered in conjunction with other symptoms, it may well militate against scheduling a case.

Tidal volume, or quantitative exchange of gases with each respiratory cycle, can be measured with such devices as a spirometer or a ventilation meter but it can be adequately estimated by an experienced eye which watches the breathing bag. The possibility of conscious deep breathing should be considered. This may result from sensation of pain and may indicate a need for more local anesthetic.

Normal adult tidal volume is in the range of 450 to 500 ml. and this will cause a marked excursion in a 2 or 3 liter breathing bag. A good practice is to use a somewhat smaller bag, yet adequately sized, to magnify the amounts of change observable.

What we really want to monitor is the degree of tissue oxygenation. If circulation, alveolar ventilation and alveolar gas exchange are normal and enough oxygen is inhaled, tissue perfusion should be adequate. A good indicator of degree of oxygenation is a bright red color of the blood. This can readily be seen during surgical procedures but even the slight amount of gingival oozing following matrix band application can be adequate to serve as an indicator. Where the blood cannot be seen directly, its color can often be judged in areas where capillaries are near the surface. Profound color changes in blood will impart a changed color to the surrounding tissues. Thus cyanosis can be visualized in the color of the nail beds and lips and the color of these areas can be virtually as reliable an evidence of hypoxia as seeing the blood directly.

Finally, the nature of the respiratory cycle should be observed. Normally there is a muscularly active inspiratory phase and a slower, passive expiratory phase followed by a slight pause. Should expiration become an active muscular effort this can signify obstruction or entrance into the excitement stage. Obstruction, when present, should be eliminated. Increasing depth, proceeding toward excitement, should be countered by lightening the anesthetic level. Agents administered intravenously cannot be withdrawn, but no more should be given. If nitrous oxide is being used, this should be lessened or stopped entirely. Normal precautionary procedures to protect a patient in the excitement stage should be instituted.

GENERAL APPEARANCE

Overall awareness of the status of a patient involves more than discrete quantitative measurements. There must be a certain "seat-of-the-pants" type of contact with the patient. How does he look? How does he feel to the touch? Does he look relaxed as per our plan or does he not?

Body temperature, which may vary somewhat during long operations, should not change appreciably during sedative management. For long anesthetics involving major surgery, particularly in children, temperature is monitored by means of a thermistor inserted into the esophagus or rectum, but for our purposes rough assessment on the basis of the feel of the skin is adequate. The use of a clinical thermometer would be a hindrance during dental treatment.

Consider these points, though. Many anesthetic agents cause vasodilation in surface vessels and this can raise the temperature of the surface, thus hastening heat loss. The belladonna drugs, atropine and scopolamine, inhibit sweating and this may tend to raise body temperature. Glucose solutions act as diuretics and may divert fluid from availability for sweating. This is another possible cause for heat retention.

Basically, the patient should appear normal. The skin should be its usual color and should be dry to the touch. Ashen complexion and beads of sweat may mean that the blood pressure has dropped or it may mean that the patient is about to vomit. If the patient is swallowing in big gulps at this time, this is a signal to get the kidney basin ready.

Alterations in the patient's appearance and feel may presage various important occurrences. Changes here may direct us to suitable avenues of investigation to determine the patient's status at the moment. Ignorance of the patient's condition is unacceptable procedure.

6 | Routes of Administration

Effective sedation requires that the circulating blood deliver an adequate concentration of drug to sensitive cerebral cells, so that absorption into the bloodstream is essential.

We can make our agents available by various means or routes of administration, each with its own characteristics, both good and bad, which may serve to make its use preferred in a given case. An understanding of the distinctive features of each avenue of introduction is essential for the rational selection of procedures.

ORAL ADMINISTRATION

Oral administration of drugs is perhaps the most common method in dental practice. Whether in liquid or solid form, the drug is swallowed by the patient. It passes down the esophagus and is absorbed into the blood after passing through the mucosal walls of the stomach or intestine.

Oral administration enjoys certain advantages, not the least of which are simplicity and convenience. The patient takes the drug himself, saving the dentist time. Drugs can be prescribed, eliminating the need for the practitioner to maintain a supply and saving him expense. No armamentarium is required. There is nothing to purchase and nothing to sterilize. Absorption, not being as rapid as with some other modes of administration, leads to less frequent or less severe manifestations of allergic sequelae. Many patients fear injections, and with oral administration none is required. Thus, a factor that might cause patients to defer or forgo treatment can be avoided.

Finally, most dentists administer drugs by the oral route mainly through custom. They avoid other modes of administration as being beyond the scope of their information and training. This accrues to the disadvantage of the dentist, who cannot therefore profit from the use of more effective modalities, and to the disadvantage of his patient, who is denied the benefits. Orally administered sedative medication has its place and much can be gained from its use, but in evaluating the treatment protocol for a given patient certain of its negative aspects should be considered.

Foremost among the disadvantages of oral administration is its dependence upon patient cooperation. He must take the medication exactly as prescribed. Adults as a rule ingest the drug in tablet or capsule form, and they probably take the proper amount. Children, on the other hand, must frequently be given liquid preparations. They often resist, either from simple uncooperativeness, fear, or objection to the taste of a given preparation and may not ingest the full dose. Generally, with sedative drugs, inadequate dosage will not produce the desired result. Even when we rely on the parent to measure accurately the amount of liquid to be given, teaspoons vary greatly in capacity.

Medications should be taken at the proper time prior to the beginning of treatment to allow for absorption and onset of effect, thus providing optimal results when they are needed. No benefit is derived from sedation produced at the wrong time. When drugs are given orally the dentist has no control over the time of administration.

Control of the ensuing level of sedation is poor. The effects are largely unpredictable because there is great individual variation in response. The generally established criteria for determining the dosage for children on the basis of age or weight are not reliable. An extremely fearful child may require a disproportionate amount of drug when compared with the hypothetical average 150-pound adult. Another disadvantage is that the time required for onset of effect after oral administration is sufficiently long to preclude observation of the result of a test dose in order to modify it as circumstances require. It is necessary to give a predetermined amount arrived at in a largely empirical manner. Control is sufficiently lacking so that deep sedation should not be attempted by this means. If a greater than anticipated result is obtained, the patient may be put into a state of hypnosis, carrying with it the maintenance problems of general anesthesia. When patients are put to sleep it is done with other routes of administration that allow more positive control. For lighter sedation, oral administration has its benefits, and even though it has limitations, it can be a valuable modality in dental practice.

RECTAL ADMINISTRATION

Rectally administered drugs are absorbed into the bloodstream through the mucosa of the rectum and lower colon. The agent most commonly is incorporated into a suppository which releases medication while melting at body temperature. However, a capsule will also melt in the rectum, and this form can sometimes be substituted for a suppository.

Rectal administration has several of the advantages of oral administration. Parents can administer suppositories or capsules themselves, thus freeing the dentist from active involvement. Also, rectal administration may be acceptable to a patient who will not allow injections. Furthermore, certain of the disadvantages of oral administration can be avoided. Taste is certainly not a factor. When the dosage is contained within a capsule or suppository, none will be spilled or otherwise wasted. However, the response is not really more reliable because absorption is quite variable, to the extent that large doses must usually be given in an attempt to counter the inadequacies of absorptive capacity. Recovery time tends to be prolonged.

Potent in-hospital preanesthetic medication, producing profound effect, frequently is given rectally when supervision by competent personnel is available. Because depression from these very large doses can cause inadequacy of respiratory exchange and relative hypotension, resuscitative equipment must be available, and supervision by laymen is out of the question. Thus, a large-dose type of administration is not the sort of procedure to be used on an outpatient basis.

As with oral administration, doses cannot be given in small amounts and increased after observing the effect obtained. Absorption is so slow, and the time required until onset of effect is so lengthy that the total dose must be estimated before administration. The adding of subsequent amounts is impractical.

Properly used, rectal administration is safe and effective in producing mild states of sedation and, in certain cases, may represent the method of choice.

INHALATION ADMINISTRATION

When administered by the inhalation route, agents gain access to the circulation through the lungs. The agents, which must be in gas or vapor form, diffuse across the membranous walls of the alveolar air sacs and are carried into the systemic circulation by the pulmonary blood flow. Because of the extremely large surface area of membrane available for absorption, and the marked blood solubility of the commonly used inhalation agents, uptake is exceedingly rapid.

Complete circulation of body blood occurs in little more than one minute. A fast-acting agent such as nitrous oxide need be exposed to only 2 or 3 circuits of the blood to obtain adequate levels for anesthetic activity at the central nervous system.

A nonreactive agent such as nitrous oxide is eliminated almost totally through the lungs. It is absorbed, transported and eliminated in its original form. No chemical change is involved. The mechanism of excretion proceeds with the same degree of rapidity as that of absorption.

The clinical result is that we can alter the blood level at will by varying the relative concentration of the constituents of the inspired gas mixture. If more depth is required, increase in mask concentration of nitrous oxide rapidly increases the anesthetic tension in the circulating blood. If excessive depth is observed, reduction of the nitrous oxide concentration in the inspired mixture, or ventilation with oxygen or air, reduces the blood level equally as fast. By virtue of these phenomena inhalation administration is the most controllable of all methods. If safety is a function of controllability, then this method is the safest.

Nitrous oxide has been used as an example because this is the agent most dentists give by inhalation, and it is being used by ever-increasing numbers. This wide acceptance is due largely to its rapidity of action and the fine control the operator can exercise over its action.

The need for patient cooperation is minimized. The time required for onset is so slight that the agent can be administered in the office at the time of treatment. In this manner sedative effect can be guaranteed at the time it is needed. The dentist retains control over the size of the dose. Depth can be altered from moment to moment, so the preoperative guesswork involved with the oral and rectal routes is avoided. There need not be fear of overdose because excessive depth can be quickly reversed. There is no offensive taste. No injection is necessary for its induction. Recovery time is the shortest of all the routes of administration; patients can leave the office in a short time with no residual sedative effect.

There are, however, negative aspects to management with inhalation analgesia. An anesthesia machine is required, which is costly. The machine takes up space in the treatment room, and whenever a mechanical apparatus is used malfunction is possible. These negative aspects represent only minor problems, however. The cost of the machine is not as great as that of much other equipment; its life is long and maintenance presents no real problems. Malfunction is rare. The machines available today are compact and do not interfere greatly with the functioning of the treatment room.

One of the few contraindications to the use of analgesia is that severely claustrophobic persons may be unable to tolerate the mask. Yet even with these patients, prior sedation administered orally or by injection often renders the mask acceptable.

Normal respiratory function is essential if inhalation administration is to be effective. Conditions such as emphysema, pulmonary edema, congestive heart failure or muscular dystrophy may contraindicate use of an inhalation regimen. These conditions, by virtue of the respiratory embarrassment they can cause, may contraindicate sedative management when delivered by the other routes as well.

INJECTION ADMINISTRATION

Sedative response, and length of latent period before effect, can usually be predicted following administration by injection. Only little patient cooperation is required because agents can be given in the office. The time of injection and the size of the dose are easily controlled. Drugs can be given so as to be effective in a single dose, thereby eliminating the need for several days' management (as is sometimes the case with oral administration). An anesthetic mask need not be used. Few patients, even those who do not tolerate an intra-oral injection, object to an injection in the arm. With concomitant use of nitrous oxide analgesia, even this infrequent objection can be avoided. There is neither taste nor odor to bother the patient. The procedure is over quickly and should be well tolerated.

Some special armamentarium is required and drugs must be kept on hand. Aseptic technique is essential and some dexterity is required. However, disposable syringes, supplied in sterile packaging, are extremely inexpensive, and no preparation is necessary beyond opening a package and loading a syringe. The number of drugs to be inventoried can be kept small, and their cost is slight.

Injections can be made in several fashions. Two types, intramuscular and intravenous, can be used for sedative techniques.

Intramuscular Injections

They are probably given more often by dentists than by other medical practitioners. Intra-oral injections of local anesthetic can qualify as intramuscular injections. With a slight change in armamentarium, the procedure is basically the same at other sites on the body. There is really no new technique to master, only a change in orientation.

A choice of sites is available, and the procedure is short and quick enough to be used with obstreperous children. With the use of disposable needles, pain is minimal. Complications at the site of injection are rare if ordinary care in asepsis is exercised.

Time required until onset of effect is predictable, but is sufficiently prolonged to preclude adjustment of the dose on the basis of the response observed. As with oral and rectal administration, dosage must be determined in advance, but unlike these routes the effect is quite predictable. Some of these disadvantages can be overcome through the use of intravenous injection.

Intravenous Injection

With skillful use of this mode of administration the degree of control can be greatly increased, almost approaching that of inhalation. Onset of effect is extremely rapid. Predetermined amounts need not be given empirically because a small test dose can be given, the effect observed and adjustments made to deepen the level. Unlike inhalation administration, the agents must be chemically degraded by the body and the level of sedation cannot be rapidly lightened. Overdosage can be avoided by careful, slow injection of small amounts, gradually bringing the patient down to the desired level. Recovery time, although longer than that following inhalation, is notably shorter than that obtained after administration by the other routes.

An added safety factor with intravenous injection is the availability of an avenue for introduction of emergency drugs should their use become necessary. In an urgent situation the venipuncture site can receive emergency drugs, and the rapidity of onset is just as pronounced as that for sedatives.

Venipuncture technique represents a special skill that must be mastered through practice. However, this capability can be attained with relative ease in a short time. As a rule dentists have a high degree of manual dexterity and routinely perform more intricate procedures.

Although special armamentarium is required, disposable, sterile intravenous administration sets are available at nominal cost. Aseptic technique is essential but poses no serious problem.

Onset of action is rapid and duration tends to be brief. While recovery is longer than that following inhalation, because it requires metabolization of drugs, it is usually rapid enough to demand vigilance so as to prevent premature emergence from the sedated state. A close watch of depth is necessary and, frequently, additional doses must be added during the course of management. Despite this, the attention required is not so great as to distract the practitioner from operative procedures.

Some local complications are possible at the venipuncture site but in normal practice they are infrequent, can usually be avoided, and are amenable to treatment.

Suitable peripheral veins are available in most patients, but occasionally there is a problem of accessibility. Care should be exercised in selection of initial patients with easily accessible veins. Uncooperative children can present impossibly difficult venipunctures, but in most adults the procedure can be accomplished.

Vein walls lack pain sensation, so the procedure can be done with relative comfort. The skin puncture is the main source of pain, but is finished quickly, and the use of nitrous oxide analgesia can eliminate even this slight discomfort.

COMBINATIONS

The various routes are frequently used in combination to supplement and synergize each other. The bad features of any given method can be masked and the good points reinforced. Local anesthesia is compatible with all the modes of sedative management and its use is virtually always indicated.

7 | Modes of Action of Sedative Drugs

Sedative agents achieve their effect by depressing the central nervous system. The quantity of a drug required to produce suitable operating conditions varies from patient to patient and, possibly, from one administration to another in the same patient. There are, however, certain constants in the action of these drugs that should be understood if the drugs are to be used effectively.

The depressant effect on brain cells must be reversible. Given proper management, including the protection of vital functions, the tissues of the central nervous system that function at diminished capacity during sedation should return to previous levels of activity upon removal of the drugs from the cerebral environment. Elimination of sedative agents depends upon the performance of other organ systems; so malfunctions, encroaching upon normal limits, may constitute a relative contraindication to the use of the drugs.

Sedative drugs act on brain cells only when delivered to them by the blood circulating in cerebral vessels. Regardless of the route of administration, agents cannot be effective until they are present in the circulating blood and are carried to the brain in sufficient quantity.

NATURE OF DEPRESSION

All areas of the central nervous system are not depressed at the same rate or with the same amount of drug. The first areas affected are the higher cortical and psychic centers, which are involved with integrative processes and abstract thought. Results produced are unconsciousness or relaxation, dissoci-ation from the surroundings and, possibly, amnesia.

The areas of the brain appear to be depressed in reverse order of phylogenetic development. The newer areas are more sensitive to depressant drugs, as they are to hypoxia. Further depression descends irregularly, skipping the medullary centers, which maintain vital functions, and proceeds to depression of the basal ganglia and then the spinal cord. Respiratory and cardiovascular function may be compromised as depression progresses to the point where it will double back and paralyze the regulating centers in the medulla. In the absence of specific drug effect on a vital center, this urgent cardiovascular depression occurs in the deeper stages of general anesthesia, corresponding to Stage IV, or medullary paralysis.

Sedative management is possible because, with proper control, we can depress selectively. The brain can be depressed and maintained in such a state without the cells of other tissues being notably affected. Sedative susceptibility of the brain is largely a functional result of its extremely rich vascular endowment.

RELATIVE VOLUME OF BLOOD FLOW

The brain is one of a group of organs (including the kidneys, liver and heart)

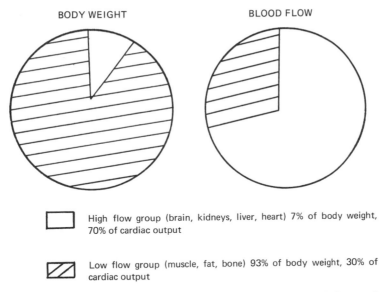

BODY WEIGHT   BLOOD FLOW

☐ High flow group (brain, kidneys, liver, heart) 7% of body weight, 70% of cardiac output

▨ Low flow group (muscle, fat, bone) 93% of body weight, 30% of cardiac output

FIG. 11. Comparison of proportionate body weight and blood flow for certain organ groups.

which, although these organs account for only 7 percent of total body weight, receive 70 percent of the cardiac output under basal conditions. The remaining 93 percent of the total body mass (mainly muscle, fat and bone) is supplied with only 30 percent of the total circulating blood.

Drugs are delivered to all tissues, but the rates of uptake and effect are determined by such factors as the rate of blood flow and the affinity for the particular agent. The most abundant blood supply is to the brain. It will absorb the drug most rapidly and should become saturated before most other body tissues. Fat, and other tissues with poorer blood flow and lower affinity, may absorb anesthetics for hours, and become saturated only after much time has elapsed.

Adipose tissue serves as an anesthetic reservoir of high capacity that fills and empties slowly, and affects the state of continued depression. Even after administration of sedatives has been stopped, a saturated fat reservoir, by releasing the agent to the bloodstream, may provide an adequate cerebral blood level to maintain depression. Conversely, if the adipose reservoir has not been saturated, it will absorb an agent from the circulating blood, lowering the circulating level and facilitating recovery. The rapid awakening following anesthesia with the ultra short-acting barbiturates is, in fact, a result of redistribution in body tissues and not from speedy detoxification. Breakdown of even the most rapidly acting barbiturates proceeds no faster than approximately 10 to 20 percent per hour.

RELATIVE BLOOD LEVELS

Sedative and anesthetic agents are carried in solution in the blood. There is no chemical combination similar to that between oxygen and hemoglobin. During induction and periods in which depth is increased, the direction of passage is from capillaries to extracellular fluid to tissue cells. In the course of maintenance, an equilibrium is established between tissue inflow and outflow and during the recovery phase; and in periods of lightening the direction is from tissue cells back to blood vessels.

The driving force behind this diffusion derives from differential concentrations. Flow is maintained in a downhill direction along with pressure gradient, always to a site of lesser concentration. As long as the level in the blood is higher than that in the tissues, the action of diffusion in this direction will continue. Even though detoxification begins, the blood level may still be increasing by continued administration at a rate more rapid than that of destruction. After reduction or cessation of administration, detoxification gradually causes the blood level to fall below that in the tissues and the direction of diffusion is reversed, with the agent leaving the site of action. Lowered drug level allows the cells to begin their return to the normal, nondepressed, preanesthetic state.

Restated, the blood level is a result of competing rates of uptake and elimination, and during induction the rate of uptake is more rapid. An equilibrium is established during maintenance with a given rate of drug administration. During recovery, elimination from the cells results from lowered blood level. With intermittent surge-type administration (drug administered from separate injections as opposed to continuous intravenous drip infusion), there are small variations and reversals in direction of diffusion from moment to moment, but an overall trend, conforming to these principles, is evident.

A third factor, besides the rate of injection and rate of detoxification, modifies the picture somewhat. This factor is a build-up of tissue reservoirs and later release from them. Until the tissues are saturated, the rate of administration is the major factor in increasing blood level and the reservoirs act as a drain on circulating concentration. After saturation, the reservoirs assume an opposite role, feeding the agent into the blood and competing with elimination. The result is a tendency to increase blood level. For this reason, injection of less agent is required to maintain a given level as the management lengthens. In fact, administration can often be discontinued before the end of a lengthy case, the outflow from the tissue reservoirs being sufficient to maintain an adequate blood level for successful sedation. Also, since the patient is not asleep and has some awareness, he recognizes the absence of pain; the psychic need for sedation is diminished. Most drug is given toward the beginning of a case and less is needed as it progresses.

ELIMINATION

All agents, regardless of their composition and properties, are conveyed by the circulating blood. At all times some of the circulating agents are being carried to and from the brain and other tissues, some are being metabolized or excreted, and some remain as a pool to continue effective action. Blood acts as a conveyor for both uptake and elimination of drugs. Removal of agents from the bloodstream is accomplished mainly by the lungs, kidneys and liver. Poor or inefficient functioning of these organs can result in delayed elimination, fostering prolonged sedative effect and delayed recovery.

Certain agents are classified as non-reactive and, after exerting their effect on central nervous system cells, are excreted unchanged by the lungs or kidneys. Nitrous oxide is a representative member of this group, being almost totally eliminated, with no change, by the lungs.

The reactive agents undergo breakdown by various chemical processes forming compounds lacking in sedative capability. These metabolites can be eliminated in the urine. The barbiturates are examples of agents that are transformed by the liver to derivatives that are not only capable of excretion by the kidneys but also lose their original pharmacological properties.

8 | Treatment Protocol

Any undertaking progresses more smoothly if a plan of action is prepared first. Architectural planning and blueprinting may well require more time than the erection of the building. Certainly, no builder would attempt to construct an edifice if all details had not been worked out in advance of construction. Materials must be ordered and slated for delivery, in correct amounts, at the proper times. Craftsmen must be hired and assigned their functions as they relate to the whole project. Foundations must be completed before steelwork can be erected, exterior walls must be applied before plastering can be done, and so forth. A myriad of loose ends must be tied together if the undertaking is to be brought to a successful completion.

There is a parallel between the foregoing illustration and dental treatment. Perhaps without realizing it, we have established routine procedures to expedite the daily operation of our offices and practices. We have instructed our auxiliary personnel in the manner of preparing materials for various procedures. It is not necessary to promulgate a modus operandi for each appointment because few patients or courses of treatment are truly unique. After establishing a treatment plan for a specific patient, the parts of the plan fit into our usual procedures and the treatment progresses on the basis of procedural sequences already delineated. How well this system works from day to day is a measure of the effectiveness of a given practice.

In treatment of sedated patients, preparation is more critical. There are several additional factors to be considered and the various aspects are more interdependent. Efficient and safe practice necessitates that each of the component requirements be met and that none be omitted. The nature of the undertaking is such that planning must be extended to include not only treatment sessions but also contact with the patient from the first examination. Appointments must necessarily be long and much time will be lost if a session must be cancelled because of some omission on the part of the dentist, the office staff or the patient who is required to extend some cooperation. During actual treatment, sedated time is precious. Preparation of the patient takes time and if extra sessions are needed productive capacity is diminished. We must never try to make time by rushing. This can lead to errors of judgment or manipulation that prolong the amount of time required to complete a course of treatment. We save time by working expeditiously in a preconceived manner, taking into account the various contingencies that may arise and preparing in advance for methods of coping with them.

The various modes of sedation, ranging from nitrous oxide analgesia to intravenous medication, differ greatly in complexity of management and in disruption of the patient's daily routine. The range of preoperative instructions and preparations varies accordingly. When analgesia is used as the sole means of sedation, little or no special preparation is necessary. Patients need not be accompanied in most cases and it is rarely necessary to require an empty stomach preoperatively. After treatment, the patient is generally as alert as before and can even be trusted to drive his own car. In the absence of certain special conditions, which will be discussed in the chapter on analgesia, medical consultation need not be sought. If premedication is to be prescribed, the situation is different, however, and certain of the following steps, to be followed with parenteral administration, must be adapted to the analgesia management. For intramuscular or intravenous cases the following regimen must be adhered to, by and large, for all cases.

PRIOR TO APPOINTMENT

A complete dental examination should be made and a treatment plan formulated. Not only should there be an operative plan but the sequence of treatment should be defined as precisely as possible. If there are questionable prognoses for parts of the plan, the patient should be so apprised. It should be explained that, with the patient in a sedated state, it is not possible to stop and discuss a particular aspect with him. It is sometimes possible, for example, when it is found that a pulp is cariously exposed and not suitable for pulp-capping, to perform some interim procedure and allow for discussion of the problem and description of alternative procedures at a later date. Definitive treatment can sometimes be delayed until a subsequent sedated session. The patient should be aware, however, that this is not always feasible and that we will exercise our best clinical judgment at the moment and do what we consider to be the best in the long run.

Needless to say, the patient should accept the treatment plan and agree to payment arrangements. Do not forget that treatment will usually be completed in fewer appointments and that financial arrangements should reflect this condition.

Before sedative medication is administered to anyone it is imperative that a determination be made as to suitability of physical status. A thorough history is mandatory. Physical examination must be made by a physician. Consultation with the patient's physician is essential in some cases and constitutes good practice in all. A written note to the physician should state that we are contemplating treatment in a specified manner and that it is our custom first to obtain a statement of medical clearance. This clearance should be in writing on the physician's stationery and be delivered to us by the patient at the treatment appointment. It is retained as part of the permanent record.

If any premedication is to be taken by the patient on the day of treatment it should be prescribed or dispensed at this time. Adequate instructions for its use should be given. It is advisable that these instructions, as well as all others, be given in written form. Experience has shown that people seldom remember most of what we tell them. If instructions are written, patients forget less.

Unlike analgesia, with deeper sedation, the patient must have *nothing* to eat or drink after midnight of the night before treatment and must have *absolutely nothing* (this emphasis is important) at all to eat or drink on the morning of treatment except prescribed medication. If a chaser is needed after administration of an oral premedicant it should be nothing but water and then only a minimal amount. There are several reasons for insisting on an empty stomach. True, the situation that exists in general anesthesia where protective reflexes are absent and vomitus can be aspirated does not apply in sedation cases. However, patients know of the empty-stomach requirement with general anesthesia and insistence on it here imparts a certain placebo effect in the minds of patients. It magnifies to them the strength of the medication and enhances their feeling of comfort in anticipating the procedure.

Another reason for insisting on an empty stomach is that patients prepared in this manner are less likely to become nauseated and/or vomit. In the event that they do vomit they have nothing to regurgitate but gastric juice which has no odor or solid matter. It is easily evacuated by the suction system and produces no unpleasantness in the treatment room.

Because of the possible discomfort to the patient resulting from prolonged abstinence from food or drink, cases are usually scheduled early in the day. If an adult patient wishes the appointment during the afternoon and has no objection to maintaining an empty stomach until that time, we need not object. An early breakfast of black coffee and one slice of toast is permissible. Children, on the other hand, become dehydrated easily and should always be treated early in the day. Do not keep a child on an empty stomach until the afternoon.

Proper attire should be described to the patient. Loose clothing with either short sleeves or no sleeves is desirable. For women, a simple blouse and skirt are best. Thus, access to the arms is provided for intramuscular or intravenous injection. For women who forget this instruction, it is good practice to keep a short-sleeved smock in the office for them to wear during treat-

ment. Men can, of course, just remove their shirts.

Makeup should be kept to a minimum. During sedation there is often much lacrimation or tearing of the eyes. It is almost certain that makeup, no matter how carefully applied, will be ruined during treatment. Also, it should be possible to observe skin color, because this is an excellent indicator of degree of oxygenation. Presence and degree of cyanosis is difficult to assess in dark-skinned Caucasians and Negroes. Yet even in such persons this can be adequately gauged by the color of the nail beds. Nail polish is contraindicated and, if present, should be removed prior to medication. Keep a bottle of nail polish remover in the office for women who do not comply with this instruction.

Hairpieces often interfere with free movement of the head and prevent proper positioning for operative access and maintenance of airway. Their use should be prohibited.

False eyelashes or contact lenses might be dislodged during treatment with subsequent corneal or conjunctival irritation. It is our duty and our responsibility to prevent injury in this manner. They should not be worn.

The patient must be accompanied by a responsible adult and be prepared to return home by private automobile or taxicab. Public mass transportation is not suitable. It is not always necessary to have the patient accompanied to the office as long as a definite understanding is made to have a responsible person arrive before the time when the patient is discharged. A nervous parent or friend in the reception room for the several hours that treatment may require is no asset to any office.

General anesthetic cases, particularly those in which endotracheal intubation will be performed, must be cancelled if there is evidence of a cold or other upper respiratory infection. To be safe, we cancel cases if there have been signs of a cold up to one week before. With sedative management the contraindication is debatable. If a case must be rescheduled it would most likely be because the clogged nasal passages prevent the inhalation of our gaseous mixture through the nose. Decongestant nose drops, which can be prescribed preoperatively or dispensed in the office, will open most nasal passages enough to allow adequate gaseous exchange. Continued flow through the nose causes a marked drying effect on the mucosa and promotes an even better exchange as the case continues.

Parents must be reminded that feelings are easily transmitted to children. It is essential that they control any tension that may be present to avoid upsetting their children.

Finally, the patient should be instructed to arrive at the office 15 to 30 minutes before the planned start of the case. Whisking an individual from reception room door to treatment room may heighten his nervousness. It is far better for him to have a few moments to sit down and compose himself before beginning the session.

DAY OF APPOINTMENT

All preparations should be completed before the patient enters the treatment room. A definite procedure should be formulated. Following a predetermined sequence insures against forgetting any part. Written checklists can save time.

Equipment

Anesthesia Machine

It is not essential that inhalation agents be included in our sedative regimen, but they usually are. The machine, when used, must be in functioning order.

We cannot administer inhalation agents if we do not have an adequate supply of them. The tanks, whether large ones at a remote location with piping to the treatment rooms or small cylinders mounted on the machine's stand, should be opened and checked for pressure. If the gauges do not read at least 40 to 50 pounds, the regulator should be adjusted to bring the pressure up. When the pressure refuses to be increased it means the tanks are depleted and must be changed for full ones.

The machine should be tried at the flow rates anticipated to be certain that these levels will actually be delivered. If small cylinders mounted on the machine are used it must be remembered that their usable time is limited. The spare tanks should be full.

The proper size and type of mask should be selected and connected to the machine. Oxygen should be flushed through the machine, reservoir bag and mask to wash them out. The machine should be situated for convenient access during administration.

Anesthesia Supplies

If an injection technique is to be employed, all agents and materials should be prepared for use before the patient is ushered into the treatment room. Syringes should be loaded with correct doses of agents labelled, laid out in sequence of use and covered. The intravenous infusion set should be connected to a solution bottle, a suitable needle attached, all air bled out of the tubing and the assembly hung up ready for use. The armboard for fixing the arm should be at hand as well as necessary tape, cut to proper lengths, alcohol sponge and tourniquet. All materials must be placed within easy arm's reach. Care should be exercised to plan the arrangement of the treatment room so we can reach everything at its moment of use without having to rely on another person to fetch for us.

Monitoring equipment must also be close at hand and prepared for use. Selection of methods for monitoring a given case depends on such factors as type of patient, agents and mode of administration we plan to use. If there is a question see Chapter 5. There is considerable variation with the various methods. For analgesia alone, for example, we would employ no anesthetic armamentaria other than the analgesia machine itself and no monitoring equipment other than our own senses.

Operative Armamentarium and Emergency Supplies

Basically, our operative armamentarium is no different from that used to perform the same procedures for a fully awake patient. Any special requirements are really a reflection of the fact that we cannot leave the patient, so we must consider all possible occurrences and prepare to meet them in advance. For example, we may be unsure, in advance, whether it will be possible to treat and retain a given tooth. Whether endodontic treatment or extraction is preferred by the patient must have been ascertained previously. During case presentation the patient should be informed of the possibilities and asked to choose an alternate procedure if our original plan does not prove feasible so, in addition to being prepared to place an amalgam filling, we must also be ready to perform pulp-capping, pulpotomy, pulp extirpation or even extraction as developments may dictate. If we extract we should be ready to suture or to perform a surgical removal.

If we contaminate an instrument, another should be ready for use. A spare suction tip should be available in case the first one becomes clogged as often happens. Availability of a roving dental assistant to bring in un-anticipated supplies eliminates, to a certain degree, our need for predicting all eventualities but this wastes time and it is better to be prepared.

The Patient

With everything in readiness we turn now to our patient.

Before beginning it is wise to reconfirm the diagnosis and treatment plan and to recheck the physical status. The physician's clearance may be several days old and some significant change may have occurred. During case presentation it should have been made clear that reexamination will be performed before treatment and that any decision by the doctor to postpone treatment for another day is in the best interests of the patient and must be final.

Check to be certain that the preoperative instructions have been carried out. Note the patient's attire, makeup, and so on. Verify that the patient is accompanied by, or has made suitable arrangements for, someone to arrive later. Ask if premedication was taken in the correct amount and at the proper time. Ask the patient *what* he had for breakfast. This often produces more revealing answers than asking *if* he had breakfast. If some food or drink has been ingested contrary to instructions a decision must be made whether to carry on as planned or to cancel. This would depend on method of sedation and the nature and amount of the food eaten.

Send the patient to the bathroom to void as much as possible. Sedated patients may occasionally be embarrassed by loss of sphincter control.

If it is your practice to obtain written consent, get it now from the patient for the procedures to be performed or for the anesthetic methods. Whether or not to do this is a moot question.

During Treatment

Administer the agents carefully according to proper procedure. Maintain contact with the patient, assessing level of sedation through use of suitable means of monitoring. Work carefully and deliberately. Take enough time not to waste it. It is understandable that there may be moments of uncertainty during your first cases but this soon gives way to a feeling of confidence. With experience we can begin to enjoy the absence of tension. By relaxing our patient we will relax ourselves.

After Treatment

Patients are never really asleep so they rouse easily at the termination of the procedure. Increments of drugs are seldom required in the latter part of treatment, so that the effects are on the wane and patients should be light enough to converse in a relatively lucid manner in a very short time. They should be allowed to sit up from the supine position of treatment in gradual fashion. Sitting up too soon can promote a feeling of dizziness. When they are relatively clearheaded and able to navigate with only minimal guidance they can be discharged to return home. Children can, of course, be carried.

Degree of sedation depends on the amount of external stimulation received by the patient. Presence in our "hostile" dental office may be stimulation enough to maintain a good appearance of being awake. When they arrive at their "safe" home, the medication may take hold again. They should be warned that they may sleep a good part of the day and that this is normal and expected. Family members should be instructed to allow the patient, if he so desires, to nap at home without disturbance. It is normal to feel tired or sleepy throughout the day.

Dietary instructions should be given as follows: The patient is to have nothing to eat or drink for two hours after treatment; if he retains water and desires to eat or drink, a light diet of soft foods and liquids may be served. Milk is better not given until the day after treatment. The soft diet is indicated to prevent masticatory pressure on a mouthful of newly placed restorations that may not have attained maximal crushing strength.

If special medications, antibiotics or analgesics, are indicated because of the operative procedures, they are not contraindicated and should be prescribed.

Minor dizziness occasionally occurs during the day but the condition resolves itself as the medication wears off.

Patients should be told that a feeling of nausea may be due to swallowing of a small amount of blood either because of surgery or because of seepage of blood from the gingiva resulting from matrix band application or restoration of subgingival cavities. The patient should receive plenty of cold, clear liquids (water, ginger ale, and so on) until the blood is brought up. Once this occurs, he will feel greatly relieved. This may not be true but it will take time, which is probably the best remedy.

Have your nurse or receptionist telephone later in the day to check progress. She should stress that this is a routine procedure of the office, since your personal interest does not end at completion of treatment. Patients should be invited to call if they have any questions. They seldom do. The routine nature of the call is underscored by the fact that the call was made by the nurse and not the doctor. The overwhelming reaction to this act of thoughtfulness is one of gratitude and can result in recommendations to other patients.

| Inhalation Apparatus

The system required for analgesia and sedation represents a relatively uncomplicated apparatus for delivering in a controlled manner inhalation agents, the components of which include sources of compressed nitrous oxide and oxygen, regulators to reduce the cylinder pressure to workable levels, flowmeters to control the volume of gas administered, a reservoir bag to provide the elasticity in the system which enables it to meet varying respiratory demands, breathing tubes and a nasal mask fitted with appropriate valves. The vaporizers for volatile liquid anesthetics and a carbon dioxide-absorbing canister often required for general anesthesia are not necessary for analgesia or sedation cases.

COMPONENT PARTS

Gas Sources

Nitrous oxide and oxygen are supplied under increased pressure in steel cylinders, the colors of which (nitrous oxide is blue, oxygen is green) are standardized in the United States by the Interstate Commerce Commission. The tanks may be attached directly to the machine or stored in some remote central supply site from which they communicate, through special plumbing, to gas outlets in each treatment room into which fit coupling devices attached to hoses on the machine.

Valves and Controls

Each cylinder is supplied with a valve on a stem that fits into a special yoke of the regulator assembly or the gas machine carriage. Modern yokes are made in conformance with the pin-indexing safety system devised by the Compressed Gas Association to prevent incorrect installation of tanks and accidental substitution of one gas for another. Pins in the yokes and corresponding holes in the cylinder valve assembly, in a unique arrangement for each gas, must match or it will be im-

possible to tighten the yoke. Since, with pin-indexed yokes, one gas cannot be substituted for another, a positive safety factor is introduced. When purchasing a machine it is wise to stipulate that it be pin-indexed.

The cylinder and yoke should be attached in a leakproof manner with the nonflammable washers supplied with the tanks. The valve should always be opened fully when in use and closed securely when the tanks are out of service. In a centrally piped system it is good practice to bleed the plumbing lines of all pressure when the system is to be out of use (i.e., each evening) so as to stress the system for as few hours as possible. A leaking fitting embedded in a wall can be wasteful over the years as the leak is virtually impossible to locate and repair.

The yoke assembly in most systems is supplied with two gauges, one showing residual pressure in the cylinder and the other reading line pressure. Oxygen is supplied as a gas under pressure which will gradually decrease as the gas is withdrawn during use so the gauge will show the amount remaining. Nitrous oxide, on the other hand, is compressed to liquid form. As long as

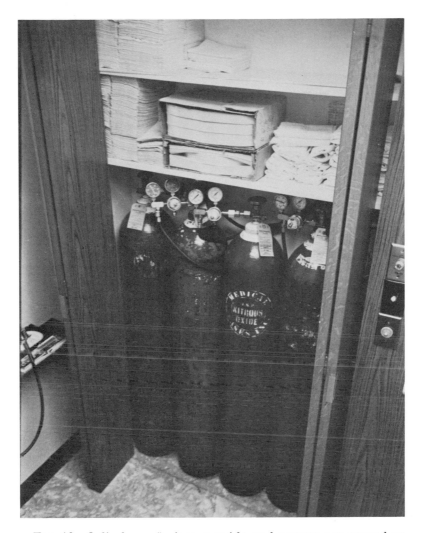

Fig. 12. Cylinders of nitrous oxide and oxygen are stored at a remote site, in this case a storage closet. Large sized cylinders are used for economy. Two pairs of cylinders are connected into the system to minimize delay and inconvenience in switching to a full tank when one empties.

any liquid remains (until the cylinder is almost empty) the vapor pressure stays nearly constant, so the gauge does not reliably indicate the amount of gas remaining. The oxygen pressure drops gradually throughout the life of the cylinder while the nitrous oxide pressure remains high almost until the cylinder is empty and then it drops relatively rapidly. The pressure of any gas enclosed in a rigid-walled container may increase with elevated temperature and this may slightly affect gauge readings but, except in extreme situations, not to any significant amount.

Regulators

The purpose of the regulator is to reduce the high cylinder pressure to a line pressure of about 40 to 50 pounds per square inch that will not

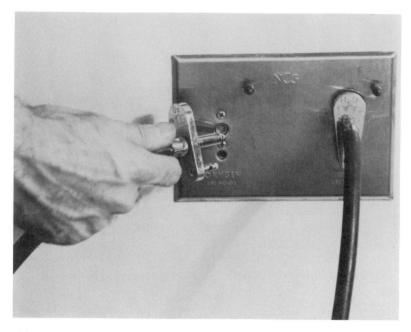

FIG. 13. In a centrally piped system, coupling devices attached to the machines can be inserted into wall outlets in each room. When disconnected, the machines can be moved from one room to another. The pins on the male couplings are of different configuration for each gas to prevent inadvertent crossing of the lines.

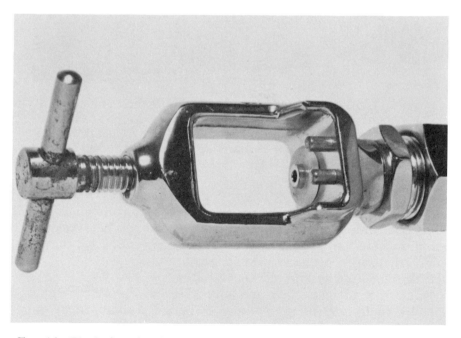

FIG. 14. Pin-indexed yoke with two pins positioned to fit into cylinder valve stem holes for only one gas.

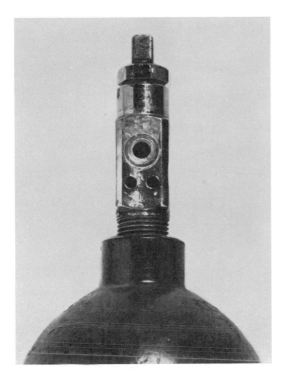

FIG. 15. Cylinder valve stem drilled with its two pin-indexing holes just below the orifice from which the gas will exit.

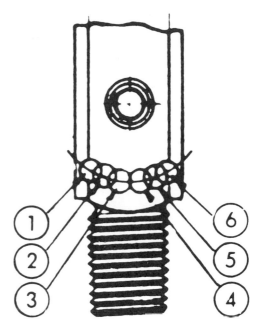

FIG. 16. Diagram showing the six possible positions for pin-index holes on the cylinder valve stem. Since each gas uses two pins, ten combinations are possible. Oxygen uses positions 2 and 5 and the pins and holes on nitrous oxide cylinders and yokes are placed at positions 3 and 5. (Courtesy Ohio Medical Products, Madison, Wisc.)

damage the more sensitive control valves of the anesthetic machine or the built-in plumbing of a centrally piped system. In most cases, a needle valve is included for adjustment of the line pressure. Many regulators are equipped with two gauges, the first indicating the gas pressure in the cylinder and the second showing the reduced line pressure, both in pounds per square inch.

Flowmeters

As differentiated from a pressure gauge, a flowmeter measures the actual quantity of gas in motion rather than the static cylinder pressure. If the flow is interrupted, the flowmeter registers zero.

The design concept of a flowmeter is simple. Gas enters a glass tube formed with a tapering lumen that grows wider from inlet to outlet and which contains a metering float. Since the tube is tapered, the space around the float increases in size as increased flow of gas causes the float to bob at a higher level, and the flow rate is proportional to the size of the space surrounding the float. The calibration mark on the tube, corresponding to liters of flow per minute, nearest the float indicates the flow rate at the moment read. Adjustment of gas flow is accomplished by means of a fine needle valve associated with each flowmeter.

Reservoir Bag

In awake analgesia management, the rubber bag on the machine serves

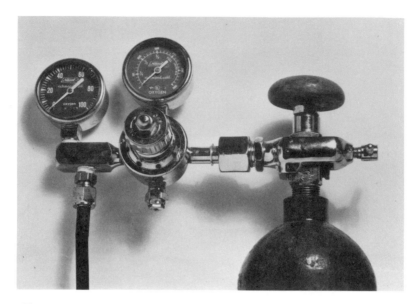

FIG. 17. The regulator assembly, with its gauges, attached to a gas cylinder. The cylinder valve allows the full cylinder pressure to exit and this can be read on the first dial (*right*). A valve located under the first gauge lowers the pressure to the 40 or 50 pounds at which machines operate. This value can be read on the second dial (*left*).

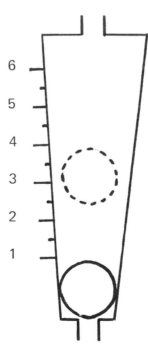

FIG. 18. Construction principle of a flowmeter. The taper of the tube allows more gas to escape as the float rises and so requires progressively greater gas flows to maintain the float at higher levels.

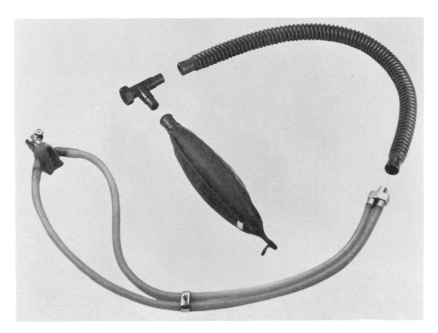

Fɪɢ. 19. The rubber goods on an analgesia machine include the reservoir bag, breathing tube (usually corrugated) and an appropriate nasal mask. (Courtesy McKesson Company, Sylvania, Ohio)

mainly as a reservoir to compensate for the variations in the patient's respiratory demands. The term rebreathing bag is better suited to describing the bag's purpose in a general anesthetic situation where some of the exhaled gas mixture is rebreathed for economy and to prevent exhaust of the gases (which may be flammable or explosive) into the room. In general anesthesia, also, manual compression of the bag may be used to facilitate assistance or control of respiration and implementation of resuscitative procedure.

During peak inspiratory effort the patient's respiratory demands may momentarily exceed the flow supplied by the machine, and the quantity of gas required to fill the deficit is drawn from the accumulation in the reservoir bag. When demands are lower, only fresh gas is inhaled and none is taken from the bag.

During expiration, a back-pressure that could impede respiratory exchange might build up in the machine if there were no distensible bag to expand and dissipate the increased pressure. A second mechanism, the expiratory (pop-off) valve, also functions to dispel the back-pressure.

Movement of the bag during alternate inflation and emptying serves as a means of monitoring respiratory exchange; this is in addition to direct observation of thoracic and abdominal movements. Bags are available in sizes ranging from 1 liter to 5 liters with the 3-liter size being most commonly used. If the tidal volume is too small to cause easily discernible movement in a 3-liter bag, a smaller size may be substituted.

Tubes and Mask

Provision must be made for delivery of the anesthetic gases to the respiratory tract. The gap between the machine and the patient is bridged by a breathing tube and connection is made to the face by means of a mask.

The tubing has a wide lumen in order to allow sufficient volume of gas flow

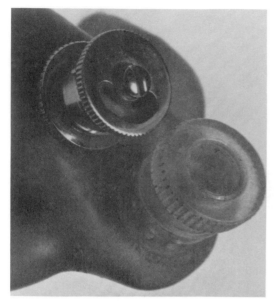

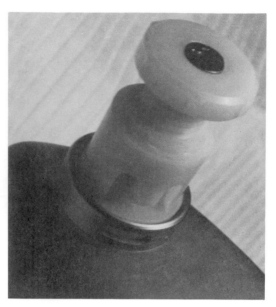

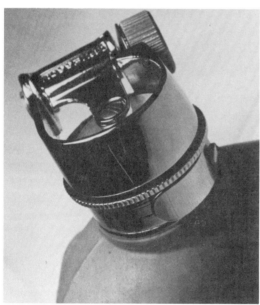

FIG. 20. Valves on nasal masks in which (A) the expiratory and inspiratory valves are separate and (B) and (C) both of these functions are incorporated into one unit.

without producing excessive pressure and is usually corrugated to prevent kinking. Masks covering only the nose are used in dentistry to facilitate introduction of gases while allowing access to the mouth. The internal volume of tubing and mask adds a small amount of dead space to the system but this is of negligible clinical significance.

Nasal masks, as usually manufactured, are equipped with two valves. The expiratory (pop-off) valve allows gas flow only out of the system with none returning. As pressure builds in the system the pop-off valve opens, allowing some gas to escape, preventing overdistention of the reservoir bag and avoiding carbon dioxide build-up in the circuit.

The inspiratory valve allows free movement of gas both into and out of the mask. With an open inspiratory valve, the anesthetic flow will be somewhat diluted and this can serve as a convenient means of lightening the level without turning away from the operative field to make a small adjustment on the flowmeters. This is an imprecise, empirical sort of method and one to be used only by an experienced operator.

ANESTHESIA MACHINES
Continuous Flow

The flowmeter machines are characterized by continuously flowing gases regardless of the respiratory pattern of the patient. Gas continues to flow

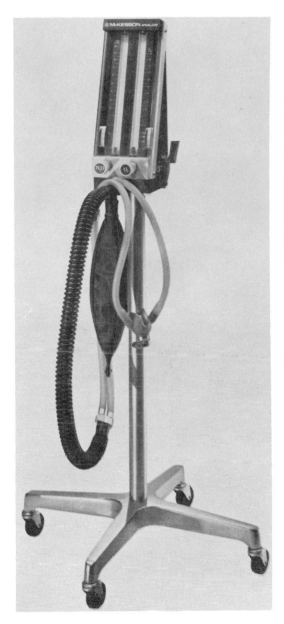

FIG. 21. A flowmeter machine mounted on a mobile floor stand intended for use with a centrally piped system. (Courtesy McKesson Company, Sylvania, Ohio)

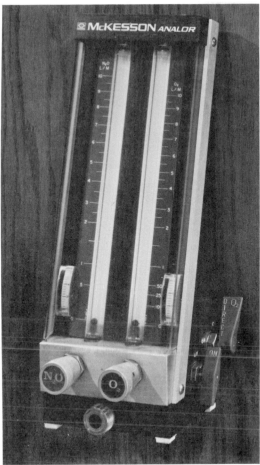

FIG. 22. A wall-mounted flowmeter machine. (Courtesy McKesson Company, Sylvania, Ohio)

even as the patient exhales and during this time the reservoir bag inflates to dissipate any excessive pressure that might be generated. During peak inspiratory effort the machine flow may be transiently inadequate to meet respiratory demands and the accumulation in the reservoir bag is drawn off to fill the deficit.

Flows of nitrous oxide and oxygen are controlled independently, each through its own flowmeter. Volume of flow is variable and subject to the same accurate control as the proportion. Some computation is necessary to relate the flows of the two gases and determine what percentage of each is actually being delivered; but the arithmetic is simple and the same figures are repeated in case after case so the procedure becomes routine and effortless.

By visualizing the position of the floats in the flowmeter columns it is possible to ascertain not only the setting of the machine but also the volume of gas actually being delivered. If the line pressure drops, so also will the flowmeter float. Checking the calibration is not an involved procedure and is within the competence of the clinician. With the setting at 3 liters per minute a 3-liter reservoir bag should fill in one minute if the flowmeter is accurate. Flowmeter machines are noted not only for their simplicity of design but also for their relative accuracy of operation.

Intermittent Flow

The so-called demand flow machines theoretically promote economy by delivering gases only on inspiration.

The gases are proportioned by the machine. Only one dial (directly reading percentages) need be adjusted to change percentages and computations are unnecessary. This is naturally a more complex mechanism than a flowmeter and, in practice, is subject to some inaccuracies. The machine shows only what it was set at and not what it actually delivers. If a discrepancy should develop between dial setting and actual flow there is no warning from the machine while the case is in progress.

The gas mixture is delivered at a pressure determined by means of a second dial. Since the gases are delivered under pressure, the patient often perceives a blowing sensation in the mask and, to some persons, this fosters a negative impression of the administration and may contribute to rejection of analgesia.

Patient Controlled

There were some machines made in the past with which the patient received the gases only when he squeezed a rubber bulb held in his hand or which continuously delivered some gases which required at certain times augmentation by the squeeze-bulb. There

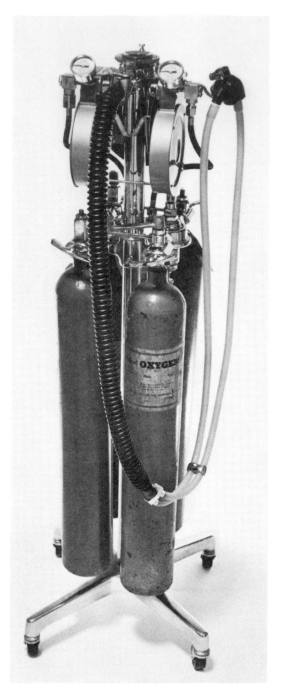

FIG. 23. An intermittent flow machine mounted on a mobile stand equipped with E type cylinders.

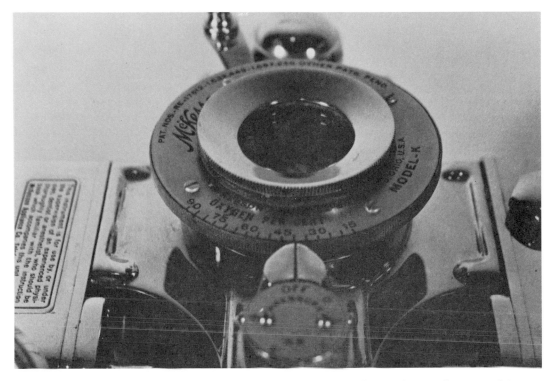

Fig. 24. Proportioning dial (*top*) on a Euthesor, intermittent flow machine reads directly in percent oxygen. The pressure dial is in the foreground.

are several disadvantages to this type of apparatus, not the least of which is the constantly varying depth which would make the administration uneven and predispose to nausea.

Telling the patient to squeeze harder or more frequently when he feels the need is to alert him to expect pain. The psychological aspects of a procedure based on expectation of pain can be disastrous to comfort and confidence. Also, the need for concentration on the part of the patient is distracting and prevents relaxation.

These machines are of historical interest only and should not be used.

Testing a New Centrally Piped System

Before using a newly installed, centrally piped system it should be tested to ascertain that it is properly made. While it is not possible to switch pin-indexed yokes or indexed connectors in wall outlets, the possibility remains that the plumber may have inadvertently crossed the lines in the walls.

For the test, open only the oxygen cylinder and plug in only the oxygen hose. Open the oxygen flowmeter and observe that gas is flowing. If the lines were crossed, nothing will come out.

Optimal line pressure is about 40 to 50 pounds per square inch. Before closing the walls and while the plumbing is still exposed, have the plumber seal the system, attach a pressure gauge to each line and test for retention of 100 pounds of pressure for a period of 2 to 3 days. Any leaks can be corrected before the system is made inaccessible. Testing at 100 pounds provides an adequate margin against the stresses of normal use.

10 | Nitrous Oxide-Oxygen Analgesia

An analgesic is a drug or agent that relieves pain or lessens perception of pain sensation without loss of consciousness. The term analgesia commonly refers to that state of altered pain reaction produced by analgesic drugs, but in dental practice it has acquired a more limited definition. Dentists use the word analgesia as an abbreviation for nitrous oxide oxygen analgesia—a form of analgesic state resulting from inhalation of nitrous oxide and oxygen within a particular range of concentrations and managed in a particular manner.

A more accurately descriptive term might be general analgesia, but this nomenclature could lead to confusion with general anesthesia because of the similar sound of the two terms. There are clinical similarities between the two modalities but to the practiced eye the differences are more apparent.

ANALGESIA DIFFERENTIATED FROM GENERAL ANESTHESIA

With a patient under the effects of either method, the general appointments of the treatment room can be the same since any anesthesia machine capable of producing general anesthesia can be used for analgesia as well.

ANALGESIA DIFFERENTIATED FROM GENERAL ANESTHESIA		
	Analgesia	General Anesthesia
Conscious	Yes	No
Responsive	Yes	No
Voluntary movement	Yes	No
Protective reflexes present	Yes	No
Local anesthetic required	Sometimes	No
Amnesia	Variable	Total
Throat pack required	No	Yes
Empty stomach required	No	Yes

A machine sold for use with analgesia might not serve for general anesthesia but a trained eye would be required to discern this difference—they are that similar. The same nasal anesthetic mask and mouth prop can be used in either technique and mixtures of nitrous oxide and oxygen are utilized for both modalities (but in different relative proportions). In analgesia these are the sole inhalational agents but in general anesthesia other agents are usually added.

State of Consciousness

The greatest difference between the two methods is that a patient receiving analgesia is conscious, while a general anesthesia patient is not. A conscious patient can cooperate with us; he is able to make voluntary movements, adjust his position in the chair, open his mouth or turn his head on command, adjust the position of the nasal mask to suit himself, and so forth. Such a patient can respond to suggestion and will have a more favorable experience if we guide him verbally into a pleasant frame of reference before he goes off in his own direction. While amnesia is variable, partial amnesia may be manifested as lack of awareness of the passage of time or of the procedures performed.

A patient undergoing general anesthesia, however, has no contact with his surroundings, is entirely unable to make voluntary movements, is oblivious to the spoken word, will not respond to suggestion or commands and exhibits total amnesia for the duration of the anesthetic period. Although it is possible to impart some training to an analgesia patient and to prepare him to accept better the procedure in the future, with general anesthesia no training is possible.

A patient under general anesthesia has traversed the analgesia and excitement stages and has emerged into Stage III (Surgical Anesthesia). The coughing, swallowing and gagging reflexes have been obtunded, and special care must be taken to prevent aspiration of vomitus or foreign matter because the patient is unable to do this for himself. In analgesia the patient is quite capable of preventing aspiration so that a throat pack is unnecessary. The patient need not have an empty stomach. The analgesia patient is able, also, to maintain the patency of his airway. Special devices such as endotracheal tubes are often required for this purpose during general anesthesia. The analgesia patient, never having reached the excitement stage, is spared exposure to a dangerous part of general anesthetic management.

Pain Perception

Under general anesethesia all pain perception is lost and no local anesthetic is needed. Under analgesia, pain perception, although altered, is still present. Local anesthesia may not be indicated as often as in the fully awake patient but it remains a part of the management in many treatment situations.

Management

Monitoring the status of the patient is much simpler during the administration of analgesia. Fewer physiological alterations are encountered than with general anesthesia so that less critical determinations need be made. Monitoring often consists of little more than asking the patient how he is.

With the patient under general anesthesia, careful attention must be directed toward the vital signs (respiration, pulse, blood pressure) and considerable interpretative skill is required. More care must be exercised in physical evaluation and selection of patients for general anesthesia than for analgesia. Possibility of adverse reaction is much greater and a background in· resuscitative procedures is mandatory. Considerably more training is required for safe general anesthetic practice than for analgesia.

Finally, recovery phenomena are different after the two modalities. Patients under general anesthesia are maintained at a more depressed level and require more time for recovery. They pass through excitement on recovery as they did during induction. Analgesia patients, however, never pass the excitement stage and do not return through it.

PHARMACOLOGY OF GASES

Nitrous Oxide

Nitrous oxide, perhaps the most commonly used of all inhalation anesthetic agents, exerts pharmacological action solely on the cells of the cerebral cortex causing depression of the nervous system. It is a true anesthetic, producing analgesia and hypnosis even in the absence of hypoxia. In normal clinical use toxic manifestations are not seen. Techniques employing deliberate oxygen restriction have been used in the past and, for this reason, some observers have erroneously concluded that it was the resultant hypoxia that produced the anesthetic effect. It should be understood that these procedures represent improper technique, should not and need never be used, and we do *not* recommend them.

Properly administered, in conjunction with physiological levels of oxygen, nitrous oxide produces mild depression of the central nervous system. The effects are exerted mainly on the cortex, so that circulatory or respiratory depression are virtually unseen and skeletal muscle relaxation is poor. It is remarkably nonallergenic and less toxic than are other inhalation anesthetic drugs.

Properties

The gas is sold as a liquid under pressure in blue, steel cylinders. To meet the standards set forth in the United States Pharmacopeia it must be at least 97 percent pure. The product usually obtained by modern purifying processes approaches 99.5 percent pure with the common impurities (nitrogen, nitrogen dioxide, ammonia, water vapor and, possibly, carbon monoxide) presenting no real therapeutic significance. Although it is nonflammable and nonexplosive, it supports combustion even in the absence of oxygen. The specific gravity (air = 1) is 1.53.

Nitrous oxide, an inorganic gas, is colorless, nonirritating to the respiratory mucosa and possesses a characteristic, faintly sweet odor; but the patient will, most likely, be more aware of the rubbery odor of the anesthetic mask than that of the gas. Nitrous oxide is stable, relatively inert and does not react with other anesthetic drugs, the metal parts of the reducing valves or the anesthesia machine. Over a prolonged period of time it may, however, become impregnated in and diffuse through the rubber fixtures of the anesthetic equipment.

Nitrous oxide is not in itself lethal when administered with 20 percent or more oxygen. While it is carried in the blood in physical solution and does not combine with hemoglobin, as does oxygen, the absence of chemically combined carriage poses no problem because blood solubility proceeds at a rate 16 times that of oxygen.

Uptake and Distribution

Nitrous oxide, as all inhalation agents, must be transported down the respiratory passages, ultimately reaching the alveolar sacs from where it diffuses into the bloodstream through the mucosal walls. The pulmonary circulation carries it away from the lungs and introduces it to the systemic circulation. Solution in blood proceeds rapidly and saturation from a given inspired concentration occurs after only three or so circuits of the blood volume through the pulmonary circulation.

Early during administration, uptake proceeds rapidly but soon slows. At the onset of administration the most highly perfused tissues (brain, heart, liver, kidneys) absorb the major portion of the gas. Because of the small mass relative to blood supply, saturation is nearly complete before 15 minutes have elapsed. The remaining body tissues (fat, muscle, connective tissue), because they receive only about 30 percent of the cardiac output, absorb only a small fraction of the nitrous oxide during this period. After saturation of the former group, the latter tissues assume a predominant role in uptake of further administered gas. Since uptake and absorption proceed so slowly in fatty tissues and others there is no well-defined reservoir to slow recovery after cessation of administration. Other factors, such as absence of need for detoxification of the agent, also contribute to the rapidity of recovery.

Equilibrium between blood and tissue levels is modified slightly by a very slow but continuous loss of nitrous oxide by diffusion through the skin, but this phenomenon accounts for only 5 to 10 ml. per minute and is not a significant factor in determining anesthetic level.

Elimination

Elimination follows a pattern that is a mirror image of that seen for uptake. A large volume is removed initially and after only a few minutes the rate is reduced sharply and continues to diminish at a low rate thereafter.

Minute traces may be present in the blood for several hours but without clinical effect.

Nitrous oxide, a nonreactive anesthetic agent, need not be metabolized in the body, being excreted, unchanged, through the lungs. When no more is being inhaled, the alveolar tension drops and the pressure gradient is reversed (as compared with the induction situation), the blood level now becoming higher than that in the alveoli. Diffusion progresses through the alveolar mucosal walls from blood to air sac; virtually all of the gas is eliminated in this manner.

Somatic Effects

Although a level of nitrous oxide develops in all body fluids, the cerebral cortex seems to be the only tissue clinically affected. The exact mechanism of action is unknown, but virtually all modalities of sensation (sight, hearing, touch and pain) can be demonstrably depressed. Memory is affected as are the abilities to concentrate or to perform various acts of intellect such as being able to work out calculations.

Since the lower centers are not markedly affected, respiration and circulation are not directly altered. Some respiratory phenomena are observed including decreased sense of smell and decreased sensitivity of the nasal, laryngeal and tracheal anatomy, thereby reducing the potential hazard of laryngospasm. The glands of the tracheobronchial tree are not stimulated to produce increased secretions as is often the case with other inhalation agents. Airway resistance and chest-wall compliance are unchanged, and any changes in respiratory pattern or depth are more likely the result of sedative relief of anxiety or approaching entrance into the excitement stage rather than a direct effect of the agent on a particular tissue.

There are no changes in heart rate or cardiac output directly attributable to nitrous oxide. The electrocardiogram remains stable and epinephrine sensitization or other evidences of myocardial irritability, occasionally seen with other agents, remain absent. In the absence of anoxia or hypercarbia the blood pressure remains stable, with perhaps only a slight drop as sedation occurs. Cutaneous venous dilation is often seen which produces some flushing or sweating. This phenomenon may facilitate venipuncture where no veins were visible before initiation of the analgesia even though the amount of dilation seen is never really great. This venous dilation might potentially affect temperature regulation but the total effect is not clinically significant because the central temperature-regulating centers are not affected. Derangements in temperature regulation sometimes seen during general anesthesia are probably due to supplemental drugs rather than to nitrous oxide.

With the small doses of nitrous oxide used for analgesia, muscle relaxation is not achieved to any great degree, as there is no direct depression of muscle contractility. However, onset of sedation and release of psychic tension may predispose to some muscular relaxation.

The cough and vomiting centers are not affected during analgesia administration. Coughing may be moderately depressed, however, as a result of the decreased sensitivity of involved tissues. Vomiting is possible during analgesia and is sometimes seen postanesthetically especially if there is anoxia or carbon dioxide retention.

Salivation is not much affected. Persistent swallowing, sometimes seen, may warn of impending vomiting or entrance of the patient into the excitement stage. Some slight decrease may be a result of the reduced psychic stimuli afforded by absence of pain.

In the absence of hypoxia, esophageal, gastric and intestinal peristalsis is not affected nor is the function of the liver, kidneys or other organs. Urine formation proceeds unaltered. Bleeding and clotting time remain normal.

Toxicity

In normal usage nitrous oxide is decidedly nontoxic. There is some evidence of depression in bone marrow and peripheral white cell counts after prolonged administration, but this has been manifest only after exceedingly lengthy administration. In the absence of hypoxia, nitrous oxide, as usually employed in dental practice, produces excellent analgesia without notably significant toxic manifestations.

Oxygen

Inclusion of oxygen in the inspired gaseous mixture, whether atmospheric air or an artificially contrived anesthetic mixture, is essential for the maintenance of life. A concentration of 20 percent oxygen, approximating that of air, is physiological and should be the minimal percentage administered under any circumstances. Certainly, for sedative management there is neither need nor justification for administering less than this amount.

Properties

Oxygen is a clear, colorless, odorless gas with a specific gravity (air = 1) of 1.105. It is supplied in green, metal cylinders under high pressures as a compressed gas. The *United States Pharmacopeia* requires purity on the order of 99.5 percent. Oxygen supports combustion and can form explosive mixtures with oil and grease under high pressure in the anesthetic equipment. For this reason the reducing valves should never be oiled and no tank should ever be opened to test for depletion unless it is connected to the circuitry.

Transport

Oxygen is required for cellular function by all body tissues, and if it is not available for any length of time, irreversible cellular damage will result. The tissues most recently developed phylogenetically (i.e., the outer layers of the gray matter of the cortex) are the most sensitive to oxygen lack.

Oxygen is transported by the blood by two mechanisms; the major portion is combined chemically with hemoglobin and a small amount is carried in the plasma in a state of physical solution. Hemoglobin, a blood protein, is carried in the red cells and functions primarily in the transport of oxygen and under some circumstances will release it. The reaction describing the relationship between oxygen and hemoglobin is reversible and can be expressed as:

$$O_2 + Hb \rightleftharpoons HbO_2$$

The relative amounts of reduced hemoglobin (Hb) and oxyhemoglobin (HbO_2) present in any given tissue site is dependent on various factors. The degree of oxygen saturation of hemoglobin varies with the oxygen tension so that in the presence of high oxygen tension more will be combined and with low tension more will be released. This behavior favors liberation of oxygen to tissues where a condition of low oxygen tension prevails.

Relatively increased acidity favors liberation of oxygen. Since carbon dioxide acts as an acid when in solution, a high carbon dioxide tension in the tissues will diminish the affinity of hemoglobin for oxygen and will facilitate relase of oxygen to the tissues. In a state of low carbon dioxide tension the reverse effect will predominate. Muscular activity raises the localized temperature, and this retards the union of oxygen and hemoglobin, promotes their dissociation, and makes more oxygen available for metabolic purposes.

The oxygen-carrying capacity of blood is closely related to the amount of hemoglobin present in the red cells. In the anemic person, where the amount of hemoglobin is reduced, the normal function of this transporting mechanism is impaired. Oxygen is also carried dissolved in blood plasma, the amount being directly proportional to the oxygen tension, but is lacking in clinical significance, as only 3 or 4 percent of the total oxygen is transported in this manner.

Hypoxia

The effects of oxygen lack, or hypoxia, depend on the amount of oxygen restriction, the rapidity of onset, duration, and the relative compensatory capacities of the organ systems. Persons with cardiac or pulmonary disease, for example, are less tolerant of oxygen deprivation.

In normal analgesia maintenance hypoxia should not occur, as blood oxygen levels tend to be higher than normal with inspiration of atmospheric air. However, the doctor's ability to recognize the presence of hypoxia is essential to proper background knowledge.

Cyanosis of the skin and mucous membranes indicates the presence of excessive amounts of reduced hemoglobin, signalling a condition of oxygen lack. A severely anemic patient lacking hemoglobin could theoretically be severely hypoxic and yet display no signs of cyanosis.

Pulse response is perhaps the most valid indicator of hypoxia. Tachycardia develops rapidly, with its degree often directly proportional to the reduction of arterial oxygen saturation. Tachycardia can be due to other causes as well; but when it occurs, oxygenation should be begun at once. Resultant slowing of pulse rate would indicate prior existence of a hypoxic state and should alert the operator to guard against its recurrence.

In a hypoxic situation systolic blood pressure may rise somewhat (diastolic pressure is less affected). But the correlation is poor and little clinical significance should be attributed to blood pressure values.

Oxygen lack acts only to depress central respiratory centers but can stimulate the chemoreceptors of the carotid and aortic bodies. Concomitant carbon dioxide build-up stimulates the medullary inspiratory center and increases both respiratory rate and depth. However, pulse variations should be given precedence in assessing the degree of hypoxia since this indicator tends to be more valid.

Other signs of hypoxia include dizziness, euphoria, exhilaration, disorientation, restlessness, incoordination, and emotional release. The signs resemble those of the excitement stage or, possibly, of alcoholic inebriation. The apparent stimulation observed initially gives way later to depression and aftereffects which may include nausea, vomiting, headache and substernal pains similar to angina.

Treatment consists of stopping the flow of anesthetic agents and oxygenation by means of large amounts of oxygen augmented by manual pressure on the breathing bag. If there are any obstructions in the airway they should be removed.

SUBJECTIVE SYMPTOMS OF ANALGESIA

Foremost of the various sensations commonly experienced by analgesia patients is an all-pervading feeling of mental and physical relaxation. The state of altered consciousness is almost invariably obvious to the patient. While he is relatively indifferent to his surroundings, he is not totally so and will respond to suggestions and instructions. Patients feel as if they are floating and drifting and sense that their reactions seem slow and lethargic. Drowsiness is accompanied by a euphoria or headiness often compared, by patients, to a mild state of alcoholic intoxication. There is usually little awareness of the passage of time (a form of amnesia) and experienced analgesia patients often can be seen to check their watches after recovery.

Subjective Symptoms
Mental and physical relaxation
Indifference to surroundings and passage of time
Lessened pain awareness
Euphoria, headiness
Drowsiness
Dreaming
Feeling of warmth
Tingling sensation
Heaviness in chest
Sounds seem distant
Feeling of vibration or spinning

There is a generalized feeling of warmth throughout the body and, frequently, a sensation of heaviness in the chest. A tingling sensation is felt very often in the fingertips, toes or lips and the sensation sometimes pervades the entire body. External stimuli —tactile, visual, auditory, olfactory or psychic—are diminished in intensity. Patients are less aware of cutaneous sensation anywhere and this is partially responsible for the marked reduction in coughing and gagging. Awareness of the surroundings recedes with lessened visual acuity so that the operating light, while appearing exceedingly bright, seems very far away. Sounds may appear to be distinct or may have a certain echoing quality, but they virtually always seem to emanate from a distant source. There usually is an ebbing and waning quality of perceived sound, imparting to it a cyclic character. The patient may sense in the ears a humming, ringing or droning. The cyclic nature of sound and the intermittent start and stop of the handpiece vibrations may merge and result in a feeling of vibration or spinning throughout the body.

Any odors perceived are invariably those of the rubber goods and they become less obtrusive as the induction progresses. There is no taste ascribed to the nitrous oxide.

Patients may dream very vividly and realistically even though they remain awake. The nature of the dream will be related to such factors as their mental state before induction, external stimuli (including pain) during management, and previous analgesia experience. There often is no postoperative memory of having dreamed while under analgesia. There may be some awareness of pain but it is usually perceived (if remembered later) as being of lesser intensity than it actually was.

OBJECTIVE SIGNS OF ANALGESIA

The patient is awake. His eyes may be open or closed. The pupils are of normal size and react normally to light. There may be some movement of the limbs but this occurs seldom, and when it does the movement is slow. The patient appears drowsy, relaxed and composed, with slow reactions and tardy responses. Speech is infrequent and tends to be thick and guttural.

Respiration remains normal and smooth with tidal volume neither diminished nor augmented. Pulse and blood pressure remain normal. If there is an apparent decrease in values as compared to the immediate preinduc-

tion period it can be attributed to a return to individual normal as a result of loss of anxiety from sedation.

Objective Signs
Patient awake
Lessened reaction to painful stimuli
Drowsy and relaxed appearance
Eye reaction and pupil size normal
Respiration normal and smooth
Pulse and blood pressure normal
Little movement of limbs
Occasional flushing of skin
Some perspiration and lacrimation
Little or no gagging or coughing

The color of the skin is usually normal but occasionally flushing of the face is seen. Perspiration and lacrimation are not uncommon. Salivary flow, while not markedly altered, may be slightly depressed.

Patients tend not to gag or resist the mouth prop, retractor or suction and seldom display a need or a desire for expectoration. There may be some reaction to painful stimuli, but of less intensity than after similar stimuli when they are fully awake.

INTRODUCTION TO PATIENT

The potential for success with analgesia can be enhanced or reduced by the method of initial presentation. While there can be some negative aspects to this technique, they should be relegated to the background in our presentation and the positive features should be presented, stressing pleasantness and effectiveness. Establishment of rapport and a feeling of confidence in the doctor and the anesthetic method probably do as much to promote success as does the nitrous oxide. Project a positive image and guide the patient into a positive frame of reference before he goes off, on his own, in the opposite direction.

Analgesia is not a panacea and should be neither thought of as such nor presented to patients as if it were. For some patients it will fail because they distrust or fear it, because they dislike the subjective sensations it produces, or because for some reason they do not respond well to the drug effect. We still have other methods of pain relief so that rejection of analgesia is not catastrophic.

Never coerce or force a patient to accept analgesia. The negative feelings engendered will remain with him and can sustain the rejection indefinitely. It is often wise to attempt only a "mental treatment" at the initial exposure with only a minor procedure being performed so that the patient can experience a successful administration and build confidence in the technique. If the patient does not wish to try analgesia, accede to his wishes. However good a method it may be, analgesia is not *the* way, it is only *a* way. Patients may become excellent analgesia subjects at some later date due to factors other than your direct salesmanship. Family members who praise analgesia, an overheard compliment from another patient for painless dentistry or that it was a pleasant experience, or dread of a particular procedure and a desire to find a way of ameliorating the anticipated anguish, may be the deciding factor in leading a patient to try analgesia, if we have not already closed the door with heavy-handed tactics that have caused an emphatic rejection.

The technique to be used is the soft sell with the approach low-keyed and relaxed. One of the key features in our presentation is the fact that analgesia is neither new nor experimental, hence it is safe. There is more leeway with a new patient than with an old one. He does not know what you have done in the past. To the new patient you just describe "a way we do it in this office."

Question simply, "How have you had your dental treatment performed before?" Patients are surprised by this approach, since they have never before been offered a choice. When they ask what choice they have, you suggest analgesia, presenting its advantages and stressing its benefits. A logical exposition would include that it is pleasant, will allow completion of dental treatment in a more efficient and expeditious manner and in a minimal number of visits which will inconvenience them or disrupt their daily routine as little as possible.

Stress that analgesia is a method of producing relaxation and not a means of producing sleep. It most emphatically is not general anesthesia because the patient will be aware of his surroundings and will not fall asleep or lose control of himself. For most patients this is the single most valid selling point. For some patients compare the feeling of analgesia with the pleasant feeling experienced after drinking a few cocktails. Explain that we can produce this euphoric feeling and maintain it but that, unlike alcohol-produced symptoms, this is under our complete control and can be terminated at will with no hangover or other unpleasant aftereffects to prevent his departure and return to his normal routine.

If the patient declines analgesia, leave a door open for reintroduction at a later date. Some persons have always received local anesthesia and see no reason to change even though it leaves them nervous and uncooperative. If this occurs you may consider presenting a compromise procedure such as continuing the analgesia for the duration of the cavity preparations or other high-speed turbine use at a reduced level of nitrous oxide and then stopping it to rely solely on the local anesthesia from that point. Stressing the procedure as an individual one to meet the needs of a given patient may foster acceptance. A lesser-of-the-evils type of presentation may succeed. We can mask the injection or injections and produce minimal analgesia symptoms, thereby avoiding objectionable experiences where possible and gaining benefits where feasible.

Some patients do not object to the actual injection but dislike the feeling of numbness that persists for hours. To these persons we can suggest the possibility of avoiding local anesthesia altogether and relying totally upon the analgesia for pain relief. This is not always possible, so a definite promise should never be made. We should, instead, present the possibility and pledge ourselves to a sincere effort towards attainment of this goal.

Whatever choice is made, and whatever method is effective, it should be prominently noted on the patient's permanent record so that the discussion need not be repeated at each appointment. Also, by seeming to remember, we tend to convince the patient of our sincerity and our concern with his importance, thereby reinforcing his confidence in us.

With children, the introduction varies little except that the parents should be included in the presentation and both parent and child should accept analgesia. Comparison with flying in space can be made. It may be advantageous to administer analgesia to the parent for his own treatment first, and to enlist him as a salesman in convincing the child. However, do not overlook the possibility that the reverse procedure, having the child convince the parent, is often successful, too. Children can be among our best analgesia patients and our best boosters.

TECHNIQUE OF ADMINISTRATION

Analgesia technique borrows from both the anesthesiologist and the hypnotist. Proper use of suggestion will make the induction much more satisfactory and effective. Since the patient remains awake he will be receptive to suggestion. In fact, a mild nitrous oxide effect will render the properly prepared patient more suggestible than he would be under other circumstances. With suggestion we can deepen the analgesic state and potentiate its benefits without resorting to increased nitrous oxide concentrations. Only with deeper analgesia does the patient begin to lose contact with his surroundings and the potential for suggestion.

If the patient enters treatment with the expectation of a successful result, the chances of success will be increased. As your use of analgesia increases, new patients will be more likely to have heard complimentary reports from other satisfied patients. Then, too, as they gain confidence in the ability and good judgment of the dentist they will become more cooperative and more receptive at each succeeding visit. Success with analgesia tends to become more pronounced as the case proceeds. The pain threshold and pain tolerance of a relaxed, confident patient can be notably elevated. Thus, success is further facilitated and positive suggestion is reinforced.

Selling ourselves to the patient is essential for establishment of rapport and confidence. The doctor must appear optimistic, projecting a personality that exudes and inspires confidence. Pessimism, nervousness and indirection can pave the way toward failure.

Since comfort of the patient is essential he should be seated with his legs uncrossed and his hands unclasped and resting gently on the arms of the chair. Constrictive clothing should be removed if possible or, at least, loosened. Since a feeling of warmth is common during analgesia, discomfort can be avoided by removal of suit jackets or sweaters. If the patient is more at ease without his shoes they can be removed. The physical surroundings of the room are important. An atmosphere of quiet is beneficial. Care should be paid to such details as adequate ventilation.

Using every approach, make only affirmative statements and never suggest any possibility of pain or discomfort. However, never deceive the patient, as a contradictory experience can negate the suggestion. Do not deny the act of injection but describe it in an innocuous manner such as comparing it with a pinch or a mosquito bite. Speak slowly and clearly in a repetitive, monotonous fashion, using words that suggest pleasure and absence of anything harmful or painful. A sensation of fatigue produced by monotony enhances the effect.

Patients are awake and can hear everything you say. Never discuss the difficulties of the case or mention aspects of the care of other patients to your assistant. With practice you will develop your own style of patter and the rapport between you and your patient will become easy and natural.

Preoperative Preparation

Before beginning the analgesia session it is wise to ascertain that all is in readiness, because leaving the patient during treatment may encourage failure. Test the anesthesia machine to confirm that the tanks are open and that gases are available in sufficient quantities to deliver the anticipated flows. A careful check should be made at the beginning of the day with only a cursory examination sufficing between patients thereafter.

Select and attach to the machine the appropriate size of nasal inhaler. If the patient objects to the odor of the rubber goods or the nitrous oxide, daub a few drops of oil of roses, peppermint or wintergreen inside the mask. Make a note to this effect in a prominent place on the patient's record. Flush out the breathing bag with oxygen by inflating and emptying it several times.

Prepare the operative armamentarium with some allowance for handling possible contingent situations that might arise. Every instrument need not be prepared, but the basic complement for the anticipated procedures should be at hand. If a mouth prop is to be used, lay it out along with a spare. Ready the suction hose with a tip attached. Prepare and place local anesthesia syringes unobtrusively (preferably covered).

The assistant should be present to function not only in the usual capacity as an extension of the operator's hands but also as a chaperone in the treatment room. Patients can dream even though awake and it is good practice to protect yourself in this manner against the imagined or hallucinated images that may cross the patient's mind while under analgesia.

Only when everything is ready should the patient be ushered into the treatment room. Give him a moment to compose himself and remove his contact lenses if he wears them. (Mask pressure against the eyes can result in corneal irritation if contact lenses are worn.) Exchange the amenities, confirm your treatment plan for the session and begin your induction.

The patient has been told the advantages of analgesia and the basic procedure to be followed. The amount of detail in the description was determined by his age, level of comprehension and his desire to listen. Some patients do not want detailed explanations and they should not be forced to hear them. Having established verbal contact with the patient by means of your greeting and, possibly, a reminder of things to come, never lose this contact during the remainder of the appointment.

Adjust the flow rates of the gases prior to placement of the mask, since with the inhaling valve closed, the patient may experience a feeling of suffocation if no gases are flowing. Such a constrictive sensation may launch the patient into a negative frame of reference and precipitate immediate rejection of analgesia. Even though the suffocating feeling may be corrected before the patient reacts overtly, a negative impression may still have been made. Overcoming this obstacle is difficult, prevention being far more effective than attempts at remediation.

Regulation of Gas Flow

The percentage of nitrous oxide in the inspired gaseous mixture necessary to produce the analgesia effect will vary with individual tolerance to the agent and such iatrogenic factors as degree of dilution of the gas mixture as it passes through the nasal and pharyngeal structures. With the patient's mouth open, as it must be, the percentage of nitrous oxide actually inhaled is greatly diluted by air. For this reason it is good practice to prevent still further dilution by keeping the mask's inhaling valve closed. With the valve closed, most adults and children will exhibit the analgesia effect at nitrous oxide flows of 20 to 30 percent. The remaining portion is, of course, oxygen, since these are the sole inhalation agents employed.

There are patients who require as little as 10 percent nitrous oxide and those for whom the level must be increased to as high as 40 or 50 percent. The most valid indicator of proper nitrous oxide level is the reaction of the patient and not what the meters read. By watching the effect produced, assess the effectiveness of the mixture inhaled and make suitable corrections as necessary.

The percentage of nitrous oxide needed for a given patient will vary from day to day but will hover around a particular value for that person. A notation should be made on his record of the optimal level so that this mixture can be set immediately upon applying the mask. When the effect is visualized, minor corrections can be made as needed.

For the introductory administration an average value, approximately 25 percent, can be used as a starting point and the analgesia management can be initiated at that level. Some teachers of analgesia recommend that the introductory administration be started at 100 percent oxygen with the nitrous oxide added gradually in 5 percent increments until the proper mixture is arrived at. This method is time-consuming and there is a definite delay in the onset of subjective symptoms which can be disconcerting to the patient. To avoid a negative first impression, we prefer starting at 25 percent nitrous oxide, showing the patient a rapid effect.

At all times, it is good practice to maintain as even a flow of gases as possible throughout the management. Bouncing around between high and low levels of nitrous oxide tends to encourage nausea and prevents maintenance of ideal working conditions. Once the best level for a patient is determined, very few if any changes need be made. Of course, attention should be paid to his reactions and if changes are indicated they should be made.

If the patient drifts too deep or too light, the percentages should be changed to the anticipated correct mixture and left at these values until new symptoms supervene. Lightening, by switching to 100 percent oxygen for a while and then establishing the new mixture can lead to the type of erratic management that encourages nausea. Conversely, deepening, if attempted too rapidly by changing to a very high level of nitrous oxide for a while before establishing the new level, can have the same deleterious effect. Changes, when they are indicated, should be made as gradually and as minimally as possible.

In the interests of economy, some practitioners administer analgesia by using a mixture of nitrous oxide and room air admitted to the mask through an open inhaling valve. This is poor practice and most emphatically to be discouraged. Since air is, at best, only 21 percent oxygen, this method further dilutes the administration of the two basic agents, control is still poorer, and oxygen is not available for flushing as it should be.

With the continuous flow (flowmeter) machines we can also vary the volume of flow of the gas mixture. For most adults the volume should be maintained at between 6 and 8 liters per minute and for children between 4 and 6 liters per minute. With the intermittent flow machines (Euthesor, Nargraf), the volume of flow is not directly controllable but a similar effect can be produced by varying the pressure setting. In most cases the pressure should be maintained between 5 and 10 mm.

If the breathing bag does not move appreciably with inhalation and exhalation, the cause should be determined. If the mask has been applied too loosely, allowing leakage around the edges, it should be tightened. If the mask pinches the nostrils closed, it should be repositioned or exchanged for a larger size. Should these procedures fail, the flow or pressure should be increased. The patient may be breathing through his mouth, and by increasing the driving force applied to the gases as they enter the nose a greater relative proportion of inspired gas will enter the nose rather than the mouth.

A patient with an exceptionally large tidal volume, by making a peak inspiration at a rate greater than the machine can deliver, will empty the breathing bag, causing it to collapse at each inhalation. This can lead to a feeling of suffocation and promote mouth-breathing. Any gas inspired through the mouth contains no nitrous oxide and will diminish the effectiveness of the analgesia. Remedying this condition requires increased volume or pressure of flow.

A breathing bag that remains overdistended indicates excessive volume (or pressure) of flow, which should be reduced or the exhaling valve opened. Usually a combination of both procedures is indicated. Thus when the bag becomes full, a back-pressure develops and the remainder of the exhaled gas volume will exhaust through the pop-off valve into the room, thereby avoiding greater pressure build-up in the anesthetic circuit. Excessive back pressure in the system should be avoided, as it impedes respiratory exchange and can produce a feeling of discomfort.

Most machines are equipped with a 3-liter breathing bag, which may be too large to allow easily visualized movement for a patient with a small tidal volume. For these persons a smaller bag should be substituted so that adequate movement to monitor respiratory activity can be seen.

The nasal masks are available in several sizes but usually only two, commonly labelled ADULT and CHILD, are necessary. The smallest size consistent with proper function should be used. While mask interference with operative vision and access is rare, the smaller the size the less likely it is to occur. The softer masks now available are preferred because they are more comfortable and tend to leave less of a pressure mark on the face after removal. Also they seem better able to adapt to the face at their edges and will usually maintain their seal even if the lips or cheeks are retracted or manipulated.

Mask Position

The mask should be placed directly over the nose and centered on the face tightly enough to prevent leakage at its edges. Leakage, resulting in a blowing in the eyes, disturbs most patients and compromises the efficacy of the administration.

The tubing should encircle the head and be positioned just below the occiput. Interference from the doughnut type of headrest found on a contour chair can be avoided by positioning the slide fastener at the side of the head so the patient will not be required to rest his head on a hard object.

Properly placed, the mask will not interfere with free movement of the head. Rotation of the head to facilitate operative access will be unimpeded and, if the patient vomits, the head can be turned to the side so that vomitus will accumulate in the cheek rather than in the throat.

Masks with extra-long tubing are designed to enable use in a contour chair with the slide fastener positioned behind the chair back, but in this arrangement the head is, in effect, tied down to the chair. Movement of the head is prevented and with the extra length of tubing, additional dead space is introduced into the system. This type of mask and this type of fixation should not be used.

Planned Psychological Approach

Borrowing, again, from hypnotists, we have found two basic patterns of verbal direction to be effective.

Predicting Subjective Symptoms

While the symptoms perceived by the patient are not identical with every administration, certain basic ones do appear reliably. If we anticipate symptoms before they occur and predict their onset, a suggestible patient will accept the fact that we are responsible for their occurrence. This imparts to the subconscious a feeling of being under the control of the hypnotist and will produce a similar effect in our dental treatment situation.

Watch the patient, note his movements and reactions, and then decide how this should be perceived by him. With practice it is possible to spot the onset of a sensation and then quickly tell him to expect it before he is certain that it is happening. Thought associations tend to become relatively slower under analgesia, thus giving just the slight time lag needed to make this work. Each time we predict something and it comes true the state of suggestion is reinforced. Therefore, when the patient rubs or flexes his fingers, tell him that his fingertips will tingle. When he moves his lips, say that they will tingle too. When he takes deep breaths, say that he will feel a heaviness in his chest and reinforce the point by placing a hand on his shoulder, pressing down while speaking and allowing the hand to linger a few minutes with a continuing gentle downward pressure. Before starting the airotor, predict that he will hear a loud noise. Before injecting a local anesthetic predict a pinch. Since, after perceiving a particular sensation he will probably remain aware of it for a while, reinforce the suggestion by repeating it several times.

Tell him to breathe deeply through his nose. With each full inhalation comes a new gust of nitrous oxide and a slight deepening of effect. This is often perceived as heightened relaxation so tell the patient that with each breath he will feel more relaxed. "With each breath you will feel a cloud of relaxation coming over you. You feel so

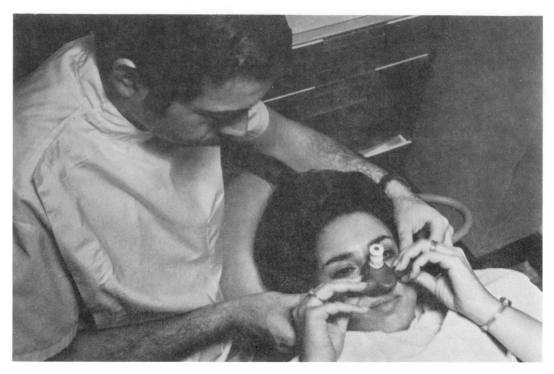

FIG. 25. Reinforce the patient's feeling of maintaining control of her situation by allowing her to place the mask herself (with your guidance (A) or (B) that of your assistant).

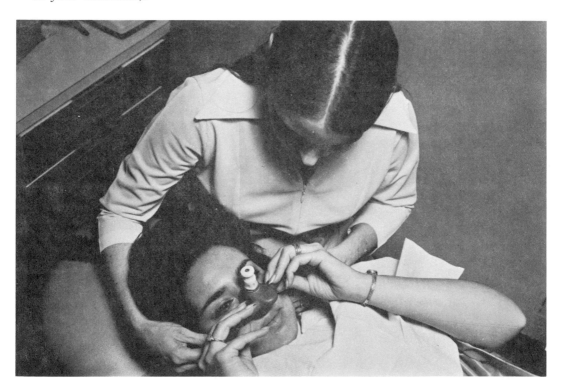

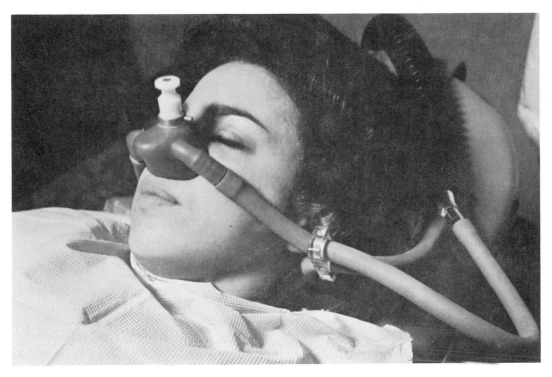

FIG. 26. When using a doughnut headrest, position the slide fastener at the side of the head so the patient is not required to rest her head on an uncomfortable, hard object and there is no interference with the mobility of the head.

good. You feel better . . . and better . . . and better. Close your eyes, if you like, and you will feel even more relaxed." Who wouldn't?

As he succumbs to the effect of the analgesia it becomes less necessary to continue the patter at the same frequency. Let him drift in his own reverie with only occasional praise or repetition of the instruction to breathe through his nose. If he drifts lighter, remind him again several times to breathe through his nose, but if he drifts too deep, stop the nasal breathing suggestions. Never tell him to breathe through his mouth. This would lighten the level but it constitutes poor practice, because crossed instructions are disconcerting, may distract the patient, and tend to spoil the effect. Make it a hard-and-fast rule never to give cross instructions.

Fantasy Picture

Certain situations are almost universally associated with pleasant, relaxing feelings. Through use of descriptive words we can guide a patient into imagining a scene that creates a feeling of warmth, relaxation and safety. With practice in delivery and choice of wording we can actually describe a scene so suggestively that the patient will imagine it so vividly as to entirely lose touch with his surroundings.

Words of action or anxiety must be omitted, since these will stimulate the central nervous system. Words describing action or rapid movement can cause muscular and mental strain and should similarly be avoided.

A situation in which he would normally experience some of the symptoms of analgesia is ideal. Probably the best and easiest fantasy situation to create for almost everyone is that of a person sunbathing on a peaceful beach where he is usually relaxed, feels warmth on his body, hears the sound of the surf (which is not unlike the aural symptoms of analgesia), and is aware of the bright sun shining on his closed eyes much as does our operating light. Of course, any imaginary situation that works is a good one.

This technique is often the best one for children who have excellent powers of imagination and are easily persuaded by techniques requiring visual imagery. Choice of language must, of course, be adjusted to the child's level of comprehension. Any routine with which the child is familiar can be effective. We can guide him through play situations. Bedtime routine may suggest onset of drowsiness. Imagining a favorite television program or cartoon show may promote pleasant associations.

The space program is a boon to analgesia, since almost every five-year-old is familiar with virtually all facets of space flight. The contour chair resembles an astronaut's couch, the nasal mask resembles a pilot's oxygen mask, and the feeling of floating that often accompanies analgesia can be likened to flying in space. We adults are also familiar with the equipment and phenomena of space flight. Aside from being a particularly effective imaginary journey it is also one that is easiest for us to describe and sustain.

The Experienced Analgesia Patient

The methods described are employed mainly at introductory sessions. Once the patient experiences analgesia he will probably have acquired a set orientation that will remain with him at subsequent sessions even if they are separated by several years. This places an extra burden upon us to make the first experience a pleasant one, because

a bad experience the first time can leave the patient disenchanted with analgesia for all time. This is no great catastrophe, however, for there are other effective methods of pain control, but displeasure is best avoided, because it may rob the person of the potential for future pleasant sessions.

The experienced analgesia patient usually requires only a few introductory remarks before he will take over for himself. In fact, he is often annoyed with our attempts at verbalization, perceiving them as distraction and an impediment to relaxation. In this situation it is best to remain quiet most of the time and devote attention to efficient operation in the most gentle manner possible. No one is above occasional praise for his behavior or passing reminders to breathe through his nose as it is indicated. With the experienced person, though, this is usually all that is required for successful management.

INDICATIONS

Use of analgesia is indicated whenever we wish to relax a patient and very few would not be included in this category. It is not unlikely that a clinician treating a person who demonstrates pain reaction will feel self-guilt and become inwardly resentful of the patient. Suffering self-recrimination for the pain he gives, the dentist can show signs of these feelings as diseases with psychosomatic overtones (e.g., headache, hypertension, ulcer and cardiac pathology). Building confidence through removal of anxiety not only allows production of better dentistry by fostering cooperation but also elevates the image of the dental profession in the eyes of the public and can be a definite factor in preserving the good health of the dentist.

While total elimination of pain is not the goal of analgesia management, this result is so closely approached for some patients as to make concomitant use of local anesthetics unnecessary. For others only the more painful procedures require local anesthetics. Thus, on occasion the patient can be spared the discomfort of feeling numb for several hours and one who is truly allergic to the local anesthetics can sometimes be spared the general anesthesia management that would be required to avoid their use. There is no special problem of management when analgesia is used together with local anesthetics, since it is compatible with all the common preparations and the epinephrine they so often contain.

For virtually all, analgesia will suffice as the sole anesthesia for many procedures that are only slightly or moderately painful. Included in this category would be trial or cementation of crowns or inlays, periodontal curettage involving hypersensitive cervical or root surfaces, change of surgical packs or dry-socket dressings, suture removal, occlusal adjustment, incision and drainage of a fluctuant swelling, extraction of loose deciduous teeth or extremely mobile periodontally involved teeth, irrigation under an inflamed pericoronal flap, shallow cavity preparations and placement of matrix bands or wedges.

Any condition caused or aggravated by psychogenic factors will be helped with analgesia. An overactive gag reflex will be controlled, thus allowing impression taking, placement of x-ray films and virtually any operative procedure. Bite registration becomes easier and the result more reliable when the mandible is relaxed and excessive salivation, often related to anxiety, can be controlled with analgesia. Head, tongue, body and limb movement frequently seen during long sessions, and almost always seen with children, can be almost totally eliminated.

Finally, analgesia is indicated for many patients simply because they like, expect, or demand its use.

ADVANTAGES

Administration of analgesia is a simple procedure easily managed by the operator and not requiring the services of an anesthetist or any other special personnel. The method is safe; control is easily achieved and undesirable side reactions are rare. The equipment required is light, portable, not bulky, and requires little upkeep or repair.

The patient is awake at all times so that special precautions to maintain vital functions and airway are unnecessary and it is not difficult to assess the status of the patient. Special preparation such as maintenance of an empty stomach, premedication, empty bladder and bowels and accompaniment by a responsible adult are usually avoided as are such adjuncts as throat packs, restraining straps and pharyngeal airways.

Being somewhat aware of his surroundings, the patient learns from his experience and, after the initial introduction, the procedure becomes routine.

Recovery is nearly always rapid and uneventful, since the effect on the central nervous system disappears within a few minutes after administration of nitrous oxide has been stopped. It is not necessary to watch the patient for a long time and there is no need for a special recovery room. There are no injurious effects on the liver, kidneys or respiratory or cardiovascular systems.

CONTRAINDICATIONS

There are no absolute medical contraindications to analgesia, but there are some conditions that tend to militate against its use even though many of these are more related to psychological reasons such as lack of rapport.

Analgesia should never be forced on anyone and when the patient shows an unusual or irrational fear of the doctor, the "gas," or the prospect of losing any degree of control over his conscious processes he would fare better if treated fully awake. It is impossible to overwhelm a patient with analgesia as it is with general anesthesia. Attempts at its use will probably fail with patients such as the mentally retarded, the severe pediatric behavior problems and those who have had previous bad anesthetic experiences or with whom rapport is lacking. Even if an obstreperous child does not violently remove the mask, he will gulp a large breath of air with each cry, diluting the inspired gas mixture to a point at which it will be ineffective. A severely claustrophobic patient may be unable to accept the mask over his face under any circumstance.

Some possible contraindications occasionally cited are actually related to hypoxia and not to nitrous oxide and if oxygen is used in sufficient concentration to prevent hypoxia, there are no physiological contraindications. The blood oxygen tension of patients breathing the commonly used analgesia mixtures is actually higher than it would be when the same persons breathe atmospheric air.

Cardiac patients, if they are ambulatory and able to pursue normal daily routine, will benefit rather than suffer not only from the high oxygen concentration used but also from the relaxation and relief from apprehension that is produced. The higher than atmospheric pressures and high oxygen concentration will make breathing easier for asthmatics and bronchitics. Analgesia management is safe for pregnant women as nitrous oxide has been used to ease the pain of labor and delivery for many years without harmful effects.

If there is a question of safety relative to some supervening physical condition, medical consultation should be sought but the ultimate judgment must be that of the dentist. Many physicians are unfamiliar with the nitrous oxide analgesia technique and may confuse it with the old-fashioned hypoxic nitrous oxide general anesthesia. They may object to its use at first, but if they will listen to an explanation of modern procedure, they can usually be convinced of its safety. However, if the physician refuses to be convinced and persists in his condemnation of analgesia it would probably be wise, for medicolegal reasons, to forgo its use.

Some conditions do militate against use of analgesia. Obstruction of the nasal respiratory passages will result in a relatively larger proportion of mouth breathing, and if the cause is enlarged tonsils and adenoids, little can be done other than to recommend their removal.

Nasal obstruction, if it is due to the congestion of a cold, can be countered by having the patient use decongestant nose drops such as neo-synephrine, and by increasing the volume of flow or pressure setting, thereby forcing more of the gases into the nasal passages. There is a drying effect caused by the gas flow that aids in opening the nasal passages and patients often breathe more easily after an analgesia session than before. There is little likelihood that infectious material will be forced further down into the respiratory system but this is a possibility as is infectious contamination of the equipment by those with colds or other respiratory diseases.

Conditions that impair respiratory function may render analgesia ineffective, as the patient may have such inadequate tidal volume as to render the administration ineffective. There is no special danger to patients with such conditions as emphysema or muscular dystrophy where respiratory function is impaired; they just cannot breathe in enough nitrous oxide to gain the analgesia effect without raising its concentration so high as to cut the oxygen level below physiological limits.

DISADVANTAGES

Basically the disadvantages of analgesia management are those inherent in any inhalation regimen. The nitrous oxide poses no special problems. There is a slight odor to the gas which might be offensive to some but this is less noticeable than that of other inhalation agents and, as mentioned, it can be masked with oil of peppermint or a perfume introduced into the mask.

One of the clinical properties of nitrous oxide is its tendency to promote nausea or vertigo which can usually be reversed by lessening or cessation of the nitrous oxide delivery. On rare occasions the patient may vomit but the occurrence represents inconvenience or unpleasantness rather than danger. Aspiration of vomitus is not a problem in the awake analgesia patient.

COMPLICATIONS

Emergencies of the life-threatening variety during administration of analgesia are virtually unheard of, but certain conditions do occur which represent a departure from the desirable course and may require remedial action.

Some patients may appear to have lost consciousness but usually the condition represents one of natural sleep rather than entrance into the third stage of surgical anesthesia. A person who is profoundly relaxed may just drift off into a state of sleep in which, just as with nocturnal sleep, all reflexes are present. Treatment can be continued without interruption and the only special consideration would be the need for a mouth prop, since the mouth

will invariably close. Coughing or gagging on material that falls back into the pharynx usually rouses the patient.

Entrance into surgical anesthesia occurs only after the patient has passed through the excitement stage. With nitrous oxide as the sole anesthetic (and particularly with the low concentrations used for analgesia), the excitement stage would be so prolonged as to make its recognition inevitable. Excitement would be marked by increased muscular movement and tonicity, respiration that is irregular in both depth and rate, possible periods of breathholding and oscillation of the eyeballs. A gradually increasing spasticity of the muscles of the arms, legs and jaw may be the first warning signs of approaching excitement with uninhibited movement and flailing of the extremities following. Dental treatment is quite impossible in this stage and there is a greatly increased tendency for nausea and vomiting to occur.

Treatment consists of lightening the level of nitrous oxide and protecting the patient from harm. Changing the gas flow to 100 percent oxygen for a while before establishing the new nitrous oxide level will lighten the patient most rapidly, but switching to the anticipated new level immediately makes for a smoother management and decreases the likelihood of producing nausea. If sufficient attention is paid to the status of the patient, warning should come early enough to facilitate avoidance of the need for crash lightening.

Excitation (as differentiated from excitement) can occur as a patient reacts to a dream he is experiencing. It is often possible to guess the content of the dream by watching the actions of the patient and to lessen the impact of the hallucinatory experience by means of verbal reassurance. The patient may not be consciously aware of the spoken

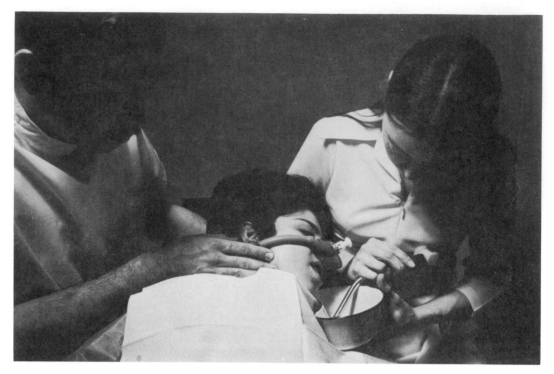

Fig. 27. When a patient vomits, turn his head to the side so that the vomitus can spill into a kidney basin or pool in the cheek from where it can be easily suctioned.

word yet may respond to positive suggestion. The limbs should be controlled to avoid bodily harm but powerful restraint should be avoided as it may be met with a stronger counterforce. A chaperone, preferably female, should be present as the content of the dreams sometimes involves sexual themes, and, to prevent embarrassment, the patient, who is often unaware of these episodes, should not be told of the occurrence.

Nausea, sometimes accompanied by vomiting, is related to such factors as depth and length of administration and the emotional state at induction. For patients who exhibit a continuing tendency to nausea, prophylactic measures should be employed and a notation made on their permanent records. Medication with the commonly available proprietary carsickness or seasickness

remedies is often helpful. Management should be as light and short as feasible with as few changes in level as possible. Use of local anesthesia will facilitate use of less nitrous oxide, possibly employing it long enough only to mask the injections.

Infrequently, nausea-prone patients will respond better if they have eaten lightly before the appointment and this possibility should be explored even though it is most often unsuccessful. If a patient is known to have a tendency to vomit, it is usually best to treat him on an empty stomach so that he has nothing to bring up but gastric juice which has no odor and can be effectively evacuated by the suction, since it contains no solid matter.

Pallor, sweating and active swallowing usually warn of impending vomit-

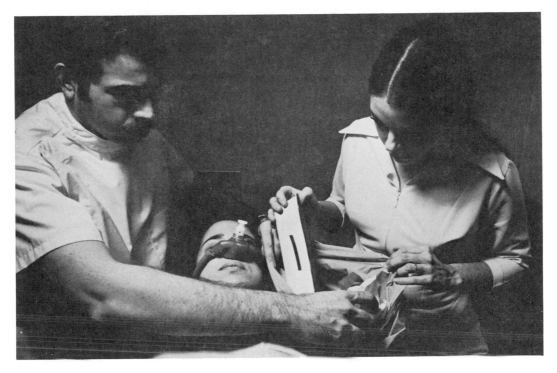

FIG. 28. Remove vomitus with paper towels and, along with the contents of the kidney basin, seal into a plastic garbage bag and dispose of it.

ing. The patient should be encouraged to bring up what he can because this usually brings relief and allows us to continue treatment. There is no special danger of aspiration as he is awake. If the attack of nausea ends quickly there is no need to lessen the flow of nitrous oxide, but if it persists the patient should be well oxygenated. In this event, the analgesic effect will be lost and prior administration of local anesthetic will prove invaluable.

When a patient is vomiting turn the head to the side so that the vomitus can spill out into a kidney basin or pool in the cheek from where it can be easily suctioned. Do all cleaning with paper towels which can be placed, along with the contents of the kidney basin, into a plastic bag such as those used in small household garbage cans. With the bag sealed, unpleasant odor can be kept to

a minimum. Aromatic spirits of ammonia, in a small pan (with an evaporating surface of about 15 to 20 square inches) when placed on the floor near the base of the dental chair will effectively deodorize the room.

Patients who have vomited may be unwilling to try analgesia again, and to prevent this, treat the episode as lightly as possible. Stress that this was an unusual occurrence and unlikely to happen again.

Cylinders of impure nitrous oxide or oxygen are rare but the possibility exists that one may find its way to your office and that this may be the cause of nausea. Certainly, if a trend develops, especially in experienced analgesia patients who do not normally become nauseated, the tanks should be suspect and new cylinders tried.

POTENTIATION

Premedication

Attainment of optimal operating conditions may require use of other means in addition to inhalation of nitrous oxide and injection of local anesthetic. Whatever the sedative program for a given patient, consider the entire administration as an integrated management beginning, perhaps, before the appointment and continuing until the final waning of effect. The dosage and methodology vary from patient to patient and must be determined individually rather than be established on a routine basis.

Premedication (perhaps better termed comedication) can be beneficial in reducing apprehension and fear, thereby rendering the patient more confident and more receptive to suggestion so that the induction proceeds more tranquilly and the entire experience is more pleasant. Other possible benefits are: elevated pain threshold, fewer or less frequent side reactions or complications, more profound amnesia and lessened salivary flow.

A patient who is basally sedated prior to analgesia administration is less likely to be disturbed by the feeling of the mask on the face, the subjective symptoms of the nitrous oxide or any other stimuli inherent in the treatment situation. While most analgesia patients require no sedative other than nitrous oxide, agents given by the other routes of administration may be necessary for success in certain cases. Conversely, analgesia with its greater controlability may be regarded as the fine tuning in sedation primarily delivered by other means.

11 | Pharmacology

The primary purpose of sedative medication is to facilitate treatment by transforming an uncooperative, anxious patient into one who is calm and receptive to our operative procedures. The goal and major focus of our attention is good dentistry. Anesthetic preoccupation is secondary, so we must employ a technique that is reliable and safe enough to direct the bulk of our attention elsewhere. Tranquility must be achieved without significantly compromising vital functions.

PURPOSES AND FUNCTIONS OF DRUGS

In clinical practice, sedative medication can benefit in other ways as well. Raising the pain threshold will aid the patient in accepting our manipulations even though local anesthesia is used throughout. Amnesia, while variable with the various drugs and with different patients, is often obtained, and this aids in gaining acceptance for further treatment and greatly enhances patient satisfaction. Undesirable occurrences can often be minimized or avoided. A sedative drug with antiemetic properties may prevent nitrous oxide-induced nausea, for example. Conditions for operative dentistry can be improved, for example, reducing salivation with a belladonna drug.

FACTORS MODIFYING DOSAGE

Selection of agents and determination of dosage are influenced mostly by our sedative goal but other factors must be considered as well. Emotional release concomitant with extreme fear and apprehension necessitates use of larger doses than for a less-concerned patient. Pain, if present before initiation of medication, produces a need for more liberal dosage. Average doses cited by manufacturers and reference texts are computed for average-sized individuals (about 150 pounds). A patient weighing 200 pounds can be expected to require more medication than someone half his size to achieve similar results. A muscular, robust patient usually must be given more than a frail person requires.

Children should be judged more on the basis of physiological or maturational development than by their chronological age. Their level of fear can be totally unrelated to their weight. Generally, the accepted rules for determining pediatric dosage on the basis of weight or age lack validity for sedative medication. Smaller, younger children, because of their lesser understanding, often require what seems to be disproportionately large doses. A fine distinction exists between the dose that will yield a successful result and one that will produce untoward depression. Immaturity of children may be reflected in the functional capacity of their organs which detoxify or eliminate the sedative agents.

Aged and chronically ill persons can present special problems that may affect drug selection or dosage determination. Aside from the natural decline of bodily functions associated with aging, we must consider the nature of disease entities present as well as possible interactions with concomitantly administered drugs. Liver disease may slow detoxification and renal disease may interfere with excretion so that plasma concentrations remain high for a prolonged time, thus increasing drug effect and slowing recovery. Distribution can be delayed and elimination retarded if insufficient cardiac function slows blood flow. Drugs that increase the work load of the heart can predispose to complications (e.g., angina pectoris, myocardial infarction). Diabetes mellitus, more common in the aged, contributes to increased vascular complications.

Antihypertensive drugs often render patients more susceptible to sedative agents. Mono-amine oxidase inhibitors, frequently employed in the treatment of hypertension, exhibit pharmacological interactions with the barbiturates and narcotics. Special care is essential as long as several weeks after such drug therapy has been terminated. Chronic corticosteroid medication depresses adrenal cortex function and lessens ability to tolerate emotional and physical stress. Use of atropine is contraindicated in the presence of glaucoma or prostatic hypertrophy. Patients with chronic bronchitis or emphysema may respond to normal doses of barbiturates with (for them) excessive respiratory depression.

For any patient, concomitant therapy with antianxiety agents, sedatives, tranquilizers or hypnotics will potentiate the action of sedative drugs we may administer. Because of this synergism or because of increased sensitivity of the central nervous system to our agents, we must reduce our doses and proceed with caution. Elderly persons and children may exhibit erratic responses to barbiturates that result in stimulation rather than sedation. Phenothiazines, too, can produce untoward

effects including hyperexcitability, impaired balance and hypotension.

Conditions elevating basal metabolic rate (fever, pain, fear, hyperthyroidism, alcoholism) necessitate use of higher doses. Conditions causing lowered metabolic rate (hypothyroidism, Addison's disease, senescence) tend to reduce dosage requirements.

A careful history is mandatory and should include questions about concurrent drug therapy, previous pharmacological experiences, habitual use of alcohol or drugs and integrity of the various organ systems. The patient may have previously exhibited idiosyncratic or hypersensitive phenomena. Previous habituation, addiction or dependence may have caused development of marked tolerance to a drug or a pharmacological group and may indicate emotional instability. There is a cross-tolerance and potentiation between alcohol and many members of the sedative-hypnotic group. Recent use of marijuana may alter response to nitrous oxide. Patients who are dependent upon drugs should be detoxified before treatment.

CHARACTERISTICS OF AN IDEAL AGENT

What the dentist wants is an agent that will ameliorate a transient mild anxiety state without depression of vital functions, possibly producing somnolence but not anesthetic sleep. The safety range should be broad enough to avoid the need for such constant monitoring that might distract from and interfere with the operative procedures. The drug should be effective after a single dose. Absorption and uptake should be rapid enough so that onset is not prolonged. The duration of effect should be long enough to allow unhurried treatment. This is an ambulatory, outpatient technique so that recovery must be rapid enough for the patient to leave the office (accompanied) after a reasonably short time.

Relaxation of skeletal muscles is desirable but not mandatory. It would be beneficial if the sedative agents were to potentiate the desirable effects of nitrous oxide without significant depressive effects on respiration or circulation. Toxicity and side reactions should be minimal. Antiemetic properties are desirable, particularly if nitrous oxide is to be used. The drug should be inexpensive and stable in solution with a suitably long shelf life.

The drug should, preferably, not be habituating or addicting. Predisposition to dependence is determined by more than the specific pharmacology of the drug. Just as side effects usually become apparent only with continued use of a drug or with higher dosages, so also does dependence usually follow only after chronic medication. In our dental treatment situation we are involved in use of a particular drug once, twice or, possibly, three times (at spaced intervals). It is highly unlikely that this will constitute sufficient exposure to produce untoward sequelae (except, possibly, specific hypersensitivity). Thus, even though we use barbiturates, narcotics and other dependence-producing drugs, we can virtually discount the probability of creating dependence. Similarly, at the dosage range employed, the side effects associated with several of the drugs will not be a problem.

SPECIFIC AGENTS

Tranquilizers have classically been described as drugs that modify the emotional and mental state of the patient, relieving anxiety and tension without lessening consciousness. Drugs which quiet and relax a person, lessening awareness of his environment, but not producing sleep are often classified as sedatives. Hypnotics are drugs that produce sleep.

These distinctions have really lost their validity in light of the properties of many agents now available. There are quite a few drugs that could produce any of these effects when their dosage and administration are carefully controlled by experienced persons. The very same drug can be used in one case for production of sleep and in another case limited to subhypnotic doses for sedation. This is not to say that all depressant drugs are interchangeable. Quite to the contrary, each possesses its own characteristics and is best used for a certain range of effect and for certain conditions.

Chlordiazepoxide (Librium)

A benzodiazepine derivative and chemically unrelated to other groups of tranquilizers, chlordiazepoxide shares with them some pharmacological properties. It excels in relieving irrational fears, anxiety and tension, produces slight skeletal muscle relaxation but lacks antiemetic, anticonvulsant, and autonomic blocking effects as well as extrapyramidal reactions. After mild dosage the patient often feels unchanged but will be better able to cope with the stresses of dental treatment and will submit more readily, remaining in a noticeably more relaxed state.

Absorption is not too rapid and peak levels appear after several hours. Plasma levels decline slowly and urinary excretion may continue for several days after the last dose. Ideally, oral management should be begun a few days before treatment and if only a single preoperative dose is given, results may not be adequate.

Adverse reactions are uncommon and usually mild. Most often they are characterized by drowsiness, ataxia and confusion. It is possible, also, to encounter nausea, constipation, skin rash, hypotension or tachycardia. Reduction of dose usually eliminates these phenomena but if it does not, the drug should be discontinued. In general, respiratory and blood pressure effects are minimal. Elderly patients are more likely to encounter ataxia and drowsiness but, even for them, these effects are rare.

With mild oral dosage, patients can be allowed to go about their normal daily routine if no unusual effects are observed. After injection it is best if the patient does not drive a car. The effects of other tranquilizers, mono-amine oxidase inhibitors and alcohol will be potentiated.

Probably the only absolute contra-indication to the use of chlordiazepoxide would be hypersensitivity to the drug, but its use should be avoided if extreme mental alertness is required by the patient or if he cannot refrain from consuming alcohol. Its use may best be avoided in pregnant or lactating women. Physical and psychological dependence are possible but unlikely in such short and mild management.

Chlordiazepoxide is recommended for oral and intramuscular use. Intramuscular injections should be made slowly and deeply within a muscle mass. Intravenous use is not recommended, as air bubbles tend to form in the diluent solution. Intramuscular injection is the preferred route, being effective after a single dose and producing a reliable effect within 15 to 30 minutes.

Chlordiazepoxide is not stable in solution and is supplied in a package containing an ampule of dry powder and an ampule of special diluent solution. Both ampules must be broken open and the solution transferred by syringe, aseptically, to the dry powder ampule. The dissolved agent can then be drawn into a syringe for prompt use.

Diazepam (Valium)

Another of the benzodiazepine group, diazepam is structurally similar to chlordiazepoxide but possesses greater potency. Like other sedatives it acts by depressing areas of the central nervous system and is notable for the indifference and amnesia it produces.

The main action is exerted upon the limbic system of the brain, blocking emotional response to external stimuli. Patients may appear alert or may drowse but seldom remember the operative procedure with any detail. Given intravenously, diazepam often produces total amnesia for the period of approximately 45 minutes that its main action lasts. Some euphoria may occur and this may last for several hours. Respiratory and cardiovascular depression of other agents may be potentiated but, when it is given alone these systems are seldom affected to any significant degree.

Side effects are similar to those of chlordiazepoxide. Drowsiness and ataxia can occur with normal doses. Constipation, double vision, headache, hypotension, skin rash, slurred speech, vertigo, nausea and confusion are possible but highly unlikely after a single moderate dose. Paradoxic reactions are possible and are characterized by restlessness, anxiety and insomnia. Impaired renal or hepatic function will alter the results.

Diazepam should not be given to persons suffering from glaucoma or convulsive disorders and should be used with caution, or not at all, for small children and pregnant women. It may potentiate central nervous system depressants and mono-amine oxidase inhibitors or other antidepressants. The toxicity is low and overdose is generally indicated by signs of central nervous system depression.

Diazepam can be administered orally, intramuscularly or intravenously with, by far, the best results obtained after intravenous use. It is an irritating drug and may cause some burning or discomfort at the injection site. Intramuscular injections should be made slowly and deeply. Intravenous injections should be made only after dilution of the drug. This poses a particular problem as a precipitate or cloudiness forms when diazepam is mixed with water, saline, intravenous fluids or many other drugs. It must be diluted only with blood. After venipuncture, and before removal of the tourniquet, several milliliters of blood are aspirated into the syringe containing the diazepam. Then the tourniquet is removed and the drug is slowly injected directly into the vein. The syringe is disconnected while the needle is left in place and the infusion is connected and started. Diazepam should not be injected into the infusion tubing, only directly into the vein.

Given intravenously, the result is usually a mildly indifferent, calm patient who is almost totally amnesic for procedures accomplished within 45 minutes. Extravasation is to be avoided as pain and irritation are possible. Given orally or intramuscularly, the effects are less pronounced but can be quite beneficial for mildly disturbed patients. It is not indicated for extremely unruly patients.

Promethazine (Phenergan)

Promethazine is a member of the phenothiazine group which affect behavior and the autonomic nervous system. They exhibit similar action but differ in degree of effect and duration. All possess antihistaminic, antiemetic and antipruritic properties. Possible extrapyramidal side effects include restlessness, random movement, muscle spasms (particularly in the head and neck), anxiety and sweating. Usually, extended medication is required before these symptoms become evident but they do infrequently occur after a single dose. Promethazine, of all the phenothiazines, produces the least frequent and least severe extrapyramidal effects.

Promethazine is a fair sedative and is often used in anesthesia as a potentiating agent to enhance the effects of other drugs and to reduce the requirements for general anesthetic agents. Its antiemetic properties are used for prophylaxis against motion sickness and this can be applied to nitrous oxide-induced nausea and vomiting. It is a potent antihistaminic (was first used for this purpose), so it might be the drug of choice for sedation of a patient with an allergic background. It is used to relieve apprehension in early labor (fetal depression is rare), so it could be indicated for mild sedation of pregnant women. Promethazine provides some prophylaxis for the swelling and trismus that often follow surgical procedures.

The hypotensive effect of other phenothiazines is lacking or minimal. Depression of the reticular activating system of the thalamus lessens emotional response and alertness. The mouth tends to be dry because of its anticholinergic activity.

Adverse effects, usually following prolonged periods of medication or large doses, include tachycardia, hypothermia, skin rash, photosensitivity, blurred vision, leukopenia and extrapyramidal symptoms. Physical dependence is not seen to any significant degree.

Care must be taken to reduce the dosages of other central nervous system depressants when given concurrently with promethazine. Patients should refrain from driving if given the drug parenterally. Irritation is encountered at intramuscular injection sites or around venipunctures if extravasation occurs. Injection should be made slowly into a large muscle mass or well within the lumen of a vein.

Promethazine can be given orally, intramuscularly or intravenously. The oral effect is mild but more pronounced than that of the benzodiazepines. The drug cannot be mixed with barbiturates as a precipitate form. Intramuscular injection must be made from separate syringes and preferably at different sites. Given intravenously, the solution should be no more concentrated than 25 mg. per ml. and injected no more rapidly than 25 mg. per minute. Promethazine is chemically compatible with meperidine and is often given with it and a belladonna drug in a single intramuscular injection. Syrups are available for oral pediatric administration.

Hydroxyzine (Atarax, Vistaril)

Hydroxyzine is a fairly rapid-acting ataractic which produces a calming effect by suppressing subcortical activity. Chemically, it resembles the antihistaminics and differs from the phenothiazine group or meprobamate. Since mental alertness is not usually obtunded, this is an excellent drug for the ambulatory patient. A slight anticholinergic, atropine-like action dries the mouth somewhat and this can facilitate operative dental procedures. Extrapyramidal side effects do not occur.

Hydroxyzine is rapidly absorbed from the gastrointestinal tract. Its antiemetic properties aid in controlling nausea and vomiting. As an antihistaminic it has been used for the treatment of allergic conditions with strong emotional implications.

The toxicity is low and any adverse reactions tend to be mild and transient. Some drowsiness can occur with thera-

peutic doses and larger amounts can precipitate tremors or other involuntary motor activity. The actions of central nervous system depressants are potentiated by hydroxyzine so dosages must be reduced. Given orally or intramuscularly, the only absolute contraindication would be specific hypersensitivity to the drug. Intramuscular injections should be made deeply within a large muscle.

Because of reports of endarteritis, thrombosis and digital gangrene, the manufacturer has withdrawn their recommendation that hydroxyzine be administered *intravenously*. The company feels that these untoward occurrences were due to inadvertent intra-arterial injection but this is only conjecture on their part. In the face of such a warning, the drug must *never* be used intravenously. Failure to heed the warning may well constitute malpractice. There was no warning against intramuscular injection and, for that purpose, hydroxyzine remains an excellent agent.

Ethinamate (Valmid)

Administered orally only, ethinamate has a remarkably short latent period before onset of effect. Most patients begin to feel the calming effects within 10 to 15 minutes after ingestion. The duration is short, too, and recovery proceeds rapidly without the residual hangover of some hypnotics. The site of action, as with the barbiturates, is the cortex.

Blood pressure, pulse and respiration are not changed to any significant degree in the usual dosage range. Respiratory depression can occur after massive doses. Mild gastrointestinal irritation can occur. Destruction in the body is rapid and complete but the principal site is unknown. Tranquility and cooperation are obtained without euphoria. Addictive liability is lacking.

Adverse reactions include mild gastrointestinal symptoms, skin rash, paradoxical excitement in children and rare cases of thrombocytopenic purpura. Adequate studies of its effects on children have not been made so pediatric use is relatively contraindicated. Alcohol and central nervous system depressants are potentiated so doses should be reduced. There are no reports of adverse effects on mother or fetus, but caution is indicated with medication of pregnant women.

With its rapid onset after oral administration, its excellent but mild quieting effects and its rapid hangover-free recovery, ethinamate is an excellent mild ambulatory sedative. Extensive preoperative preparations are not necessary. The drug can be given right at the time of treatment should the need for some mild sedation become apparent.

Meprobamate (Equanil, Miltown)

Meprobamate is an effective ataractic for relieving moderate tension and anxiety but lacks potency for more severe cases. It exerts a depressant effect on the limbic system, thalamus and basal ganglia without affecting the cerebral cortex. Autonomic and antihistaminic effects are lacking. The usual clinical picture is one of reduced anxiety, excitability and muscular tension with lessened responses to stressful stimuli. It is not an hypnotic specifically, but relief of anxiety often makes normal sleep possible. Ninety percent is metabolized by conjugation and ten percent is excreted unchanged in the urine.

The overall toxicity is low. Drowsiness and mild ataxia are the most commonly seen reactions. Physical and psychic dependence can occur after prolonged therapy with the possibility of withdrawal symptoms following abrupt cessation. Paradoxic reaction

characterized by excitement, abdominal cramping, diarrhea and muscular hypertonicity can occur but is rare. The most common side reactions include erythematous skin eruptions, itching, angioneurotic edema, fever, double vision, hypotension, vertigo and drowsiness. Allergy or idiosyncrasy are rare. Tolerance can develop to sustained therapy.

Normal therapeutic dosage usually will not impair reaction time or depth perception, so driving is not contraindicated (unless drowsiness is apparent). Seizures might occasionally be precipitated in epileptic patients and there is a synergism with alcohol and other central nervous system depressants. Meprobamate passes the placental barrier and safe use in pregnancy is not definitely established.

Meprobamate is available usually in tablet form. The tablets are large but should be swallowed whole rather than chewed, as they have a rather unpleasant taste. There is some latitude in dosage as long as impaired alertness is not apparent. A sustained release tablet is available. Intravenous administration is contraindicated, as thrombosis and hemolysis have been known to occur.

Short-Acting Barbiturates—Secobarbital (Seconal) and Pentobarbital (Nembutal)

Barbiturates act primarily by preventing impulses in the ascending reticular formation from being transmitted to the cerebral cortex, but they also directly depress cells in cortical sensory and motor areas. The resultant effect can range from mild sedation through hypnosis to general anesthesia depending upon the particular barbiturate used, its dose, the route of administration and the patient's level of reflex excitability.

Barbiturates are classified according to their duration of action from ultrashort to long. The shorter acting drugs have correspondingly shorter onset times and generally exert more profound depression. Choice of drug must be made on the basis of the requirements of the specific case and the desired method of administration. Often, several drugs can be used for the same result. We recommend secobarbital and pentobarbital for the technique described here.

In subhypnotic doses, barbiturates produce few side effects. Sleep, when it occurs, resembles a dreamless natural sleep but a hangover can persist for several hours after awakening. In larger doses barbiturates are potent depressors of the respiratory and vasomotor centers.

Pain is not significantly obtunded until quite intense depression has occurred. In subhypnotic doses, the pain threshold may be lowered. Hypnotic doses may produce delirium rather than sleep in the presence of moderate to severe pain. And yet, the barbiturates definitely potentiate the effects of analgesic drugs.

Ordinary sedative and hypnotic doses do not significantly affect cardiovascular function. A slight fall in blood pressure and pulse at the beginning of the case probably represents a return to an unanxious base line rather than depression and is more desirable than not. Rapid intravenous injection, or large doses by any route, depress the vasomotor center causing peripheral vasodilation and hypotension which return to normal as the drug is eliminated.

Therapeutic doses have little effect on respiration but larger doses, particularly if given intravenously, depress the respiratory center in the medulla reducing its responsiveness to carbon dioxide. Pulmonary ventilation is reduced as depth and rate diminish. Death, when it occurs from barbiturate poisoning, is usually due to respiratory failure. Doses approaching the hypnotic range may predispose to laryngeal or pharyngeal spasm.

Barbiturates are readily absorbed from the stomach, small intestine, rectum, muscle and subcutaneous tissue. They are distributed to all the tissues of the body and cross the placental barrier but exert their depressive action only on the brain. The relative concentration in different tissues depends on local blood supply. Brain, liver and kidney, having proportionately greater blood supply per unit mass, receive relatively more drug while bone and muscle get less. Reservoirs in body fat become saturated after some time and it is the withdrawal of agent from blood to these repositories that accounts for the rapid recovery of some barbiturates. Even the shortest acting barbiturates are metabolized no faster than 15 percent per hour so emergence is more a factor of redistribution than of breakdown or excretion. The shorter acting barbiturates are broken down mainly in the liver while the longer acting ones are excreted mostly unchanged by the kidneys.

Toxicity is low in therapeutic doses to normal persons. Paradoxic reactions causing excitement, restlessness and delirium can occur in children and the elderly. There is a low incidence of allergy, skin rash and gastrointestinal symptoms. A synergism causing sudden severe depression can result from concurrent use of alcohol, antihistamines or reserpine. Acute toxicity from overdose is manifested mainly as respiratory depression. Tolerance can result from chronic use. Aqueous solutions of barbiturates are highly alkaline and extravasation around a venipuncture can cause thrombophlebitis or tissue necrosis. Dilution of the drug by injection into the tubing of an intravenous infusion lessens the incidence of these complications.

Short-acting barbiturates should not be used for persons suffering from liver disease. Similarly, renal disease contra-indicates use of the longer acting members of the group. Some psychoneurotic persons respond with restlessness and confusion. Idiosyncrasy or previous habituation are contraindicating factors. Problems may develop after administration to persons with hyperthyroidism, diabetes mellitus, severe anemia or congestive heart failure.

Given orally or intramuscularly, secobarbital is noticeably shorter acting than pentobarbital. The recovery time of the latter is sufficiently prolonged to negate its benefits for ambulatory management. With intravenous use this distinction becomes less clear. While secobarbital remains shorter acting, the onset and action of pentobarbital becomes shorter and the two agents are almost interchangeable. For cases under an hour, secobarbital is preferred. As the anticipated duration exceeds one hour, pentobarbital becomes the more likely choice. Whichever drug was used initially, further injections as the case progresses are best made with secobarbital. After use of either agent, the patient's alertness will be impaired for several hours. He should be discharged only in the company of a responsible adult and prohibited from driving for the remainder of the day. After arriving home he will probably sleep for several hours and family members should be advised of this and instructed not to disturb him.

Because of the irritating alkalinity of these drugs, intramuscular injections should be made deeply into a large muscle with not more than 5 ml. injected at any one site regardless of dilution. Intravenous injection should be made no more rapidly than 25 mg. per 15 seconds. Concomitantly administered drugs should be considered on the basis of synergizing potential and the dosages of all agents reduced accordingly.

Chloral Hydrate (Noctec)

One of the oldest members of the hypnotic group, chloral hydrate, a chlorinated derivative of ethyl alcohol, was first synthesized in 1832. In contrast to the barbiturates, it has less potential for habituation, paradoxic reaction, tolerance and hangover and depresses motor activity to some extent. Analgesia is similarly lacking. It is known for its characteristic penetrating odor and bitter taste but these have been effectively masked in currently available syrups. Taken orally, drowsiness can occur within 20 minutes and can last as long as 5 to 8 hours.

In therapeutic doses the effects are limited to the cerebral hemispheres with the medullary vital centers remaining unaffected. In healthy patients, blood pressure and respiration are little more depressed than by ordinary sleep. Dangerous depression usually occurs only after toxic doses.

Chloral hydrate is readily absorbed from the gastrointestinal tract but tends to irritate the gastric mucosa causing nausea and vomiting. It is converted in the liver to trichloroacetic acid and trichloroethanol (which actually produces the sleep). The metabolites are excreted by the kidneys. Presence of kidney or liver disease are indications for medical consultation prior to use.

Use of chloral hydrate is contraindicated for patients suffering from peptic or duodenal ulcer, chronic indigestion or from serious heart, liver or kidney disease. Tolerance stems from an increased capacity of the liver to break it down. Habituation is not common but can occur after repeated dosages. In normal use, this is an agent that is characterized by a wide safety margin and freedom from side effects. It is usually considered safe for children and the elderly, for whom barbiturates may be relatively contraindicated. The symptoms of acute poisoning include deep stupor, marked peripheral vasodilation, hypotension, slow respiration, hypothermia and, occasionally, delirium. If untreated, death can occur from respiratory depression or from cardiac collapse in patients with impaired heart function. Profound synergism exists between chloral hydrate and alcohol (knockout drops, Mickey Finn).

In clinical use the sedative effects are variable. Some children may drowse; others may exhibit only some ataxia. In the dental chair they all revive to some degree but when nitrous oxide analgesia is added to the management, results are almost universally successful. The patient usually falls asleep on the way home and tends to sleep peacefully for several hours. The potential for nausea and vomiting have been largely overcome by dispensing the chloral hydrate mixed with promethazine. (See oral administration, p. 113.)

Meperidine (Demerol)

The main action of meperidine, a synthetic narcotic, is to depress cerebral response to pain but some sedation occurs too. The analgesic potency is less than that of morphine but greater than that of codeine. The sedative action must usually be potentiated by other agents for truly effective results. Meperidine, in turn, potentiates the sleep-producing capability of barbiturates and other hypnotics while adding analgesic properties to the mixture.

The major effect is on the central nervous system but the exact mechanism of action is unknown. Usual doses produce analgesia plus some euphoria and sedation. Hypnosis occurs with larger doses. The sleep produced tends to be of short duration and the patient is easily roused. Doses above the therapeutic range tend to excite rather than depress further.

Respiration can be seriously depressed by toxic doses but is little affected in the therapeutic range. Depression is usually seen more in rate than depth and is more common after intravenous administration. Respiratory depression tends to be transient and is reversed by the narcotic antagonists nalorphine (Nalline) and levallorphan (Lorfan). Unlike codeine, the cough reflex is not depressed.

Cardiovascular effects are mild if the patient is in a recumbent position but may tend to lowering of blood pressure if the patient remains upright. A small percentage of patients may show syncope-like hypotension and bradycardia. Intravenous administration provokes a greater incidence of such occurrences but of a transient nature.

Meperidine is rapidly absorbed after both oral and parenteral administration. The liver metabolizes approximately 90 percent with the remainder excreted in the urine along with its degradation products. Persons with liver disease will show an exaggerated response.

Adverse reactions after mild to moderate doses tend to be of a transitory nature but are more frequent after intravenous injection or ambulation too soon after administration. Possible symptoms include weakness, vertigo, nausea, vomiting, sweating, visual disturbances, respiratory depression, blurred vision, fainting and, rarely, urticaria. Overdose can cause cerebral excitation with tremors and muscular incoordination. Precipitous blood pressure drop is possible if given to patients on mono-amine oxidase inhibitors. The constipation and urinary retention often seen after use of other opiates does not occur with meperidine. Tolerance, habituation and addiction can occur after chronic use.

Use of meperidine is not specifically contraindicated by any disease entity except liver dysfunction or intracranial pressure. Special caution is required with hypothyroidism or adrenal cortical insufficiency. Intravenous injection should be made slowly in divided doses to avoid a hypotensive reaction.

A very commonly used clinical method of enhancing the sedative propensity of meperidine is by combination with promethazine. The two drugs are compatible and can be mixed in a single syringe for intramuscular injection but should be given separately when injected intravenously. When combined for intramuscular administration, the total volume of solution should be kept as small as possible to minimize post-injection soreness at the site.

Alphaprodine (Nisentil)

Chemically similar to meperidine, alphaprodine shares the same pharmacological properties as the rest of the synthetic nonopiate analgesics. Its analgesia is slightly more potent than that of meperidine. Its onset is more rapid and its duration shorter.

Alphaprodine's pharmacological properties, toxicity, adverse reactions and contraindications resemble those cited for meperidine. Nausea and vomiting are less commonly seen than with some of the narcotics. Tolerance and addiction may develop.

Since we are dealing with ambulatory patients, the shorter duration of alphaprodine is an indication for its use. Combination with a narcotic antagonist theoretically counters any potential respiratory depression without lessening the analgesic potency of the narcotic, if the therapeutic mixture is made in the proper ratio.

Levallorphan (Lorfan)

The respiratory depressant effects of the narcotics can theoretically be abolished by use of the narcotic antagonists nalorphine (Nalline) or levallorphan (Lorfan). These drugs are used, together with supportive measures, in the treatment of the respiratory depression of acute narcotic poisoning. Both respiratory rate and minute volume will be increased. The prompt reversal can be lifesaving. In this application, however, they often reduce or nullify the analgesic or sedative effects as well.

Curiously, if an antagonist is given to an unnarcotized individual, it will, itself, depress respiration. Similarly, if the antagonist is of longer duration than the narcotic, depression will occur after the narcotic wears off. If the antagonist is of shorter duration than the narcotic, respiratory depression can result when the antagonist wears off. If the dosage of the antagonist is too great relative to that of the narcotic, the analgesia may be lost.

In sedative management we wish only to counter the respiratory effects of the narcotic without lessening its sedative analgesia. This is accomplished by using a drug from each group with similar duration of action and by carefully regulating their ratio. Levallorphan and alphaprodine are matched because their durations are short enough for outpatient management and similar in length. The optimum ratio is 50 parts of alphaprodine to 1 part of levallorphan. (See intravenous administration, p. 146.)

Atropine

Now prepared synthetically, atropine was originally extracted from belladonna plants. Its most important action is an inhibition of effector organs (especially those containing smooth muscle or secretory glands) innervated by postganglionic cholinergic nerves. Cerebral effect varies according to dosage. In anesthesia it is used to reduce salivary and bronchial secretions and as prophylaxis against vagal reflexes that can cause laryngeal spasm.

The parasympatholytic effect results from blocking the action of acetylcholine at effector cells or neuromuscular junctions of organs innervated by postganglionic cholinergic nerves. The effects produced are similar to those seen when epinephrine is given or the sympathetic nervous system is otherwise stimulated. Atropine neither destroys nor prevents the formation of acetylcholine. It merely competes for its sites on effector cells.

The central nervous system is first stimulated with small doses and then depressed as toxic amounts are approached. Very large doses can cause hallucinations, restlessness and delirium.

The primary effect on the heart is to alter its rate. Depression of vagal tone quickens the pulse. Vagal tone is greater in young persons so they show a more profound effect. Larger doses dilate cutaneous vessels and, with toxic doses, central vasomotor depression can decrease the blood pressure.

The medullary respiratory center is stimulated by clinical doses so respiration becomes deeper and more rapid. Mucous membranes become dry as glandular secretions are inhibited. The bronchi and bronchioles dilate as their smooth muscle relaxes.

Secretion of tears, sweat, saliva and gastric juice are lessened as their glands are inhibited. The skin becomes warm and dry and body temperature may rise with large doses. The pupils of the eyes are dilated and unresponsive to light, while the lenses become fixed for far vision.

The classic signs of an atropinized patient are dry mouth and nose, thirst, flushing of the face and neck, dry skin, rapid heart, urinary retention, dilated pupils and blurred vision.

Atropine is rapidly absorbed and distributed throughout the body. Most of it is hydrolyzed by enzymes in the liver. A small amount is excreted unchanged in the urine.

Its use is contraindicated for patients with glaucoma, prostatic hypertrophy and asthma and, because of the possible tachycardia, relatively contraindicated in the presence of cardiovascular disease. Generally, it should not be given to patients older than forty years.

Whether prophylaxis against vagal reflexes is truly accomplished with the usual dose of 0.4 to 0.5 mg. is subject to some debate. Similarly, the need for salivary depression for operative dentistry may be overemphasized. It has been our experience that, in a lengthy operative case, dryness (even without atropine) is more apparent than salivary excess and that atropine is not necessary.

12 | Oral Administration

Ingestion of the drug by mouth is undoubtedly the most commonly used method for administration of sedatives in dental practice. After passing down the esophagus, the drug passes through the mucosal walls of the stomach or intestine and is absorbed into the bloodstream.

ADVANTAGES

Of all the routes of administration, this is the simplest and most convenient. The drug can be prescribed for the patient to take himself, thereby saving time in the office. No special armamentarium need be purchased or sterilized, and the dentist need not maintain an inventory of these drugs. Savings accrue in time, effort and expense.

Fearful patients may not be able to accept a mask on the face or injection of either local anesthetics in the mouth or sedative agents into the arm or elsewhere. However, very few persons object to swallowing medication (in the proper dosage form), and this can serve as an introductory method to calm the patient sufficiently so that he will accept the other procedures. Even claustrophobes who would never ordinarily tolerate a mask over the face usually submit docilely after light orally administered sedation. For other patients who fear intramuscular or intravenous injections or the analgesia mask, oral sedation is similarly beneficial. In still other cases, oral sedation serves not just as an introductory process, facilitating use of these other modalities, but is rather a substitute by itself, producing a state in which dental treatment can be accomplished.

Since absorption of medication through the gastric and intestinal mucosa proceeds slowly, allergic manifestations tend to be less severe. further, the duration of sedative action tends to be prolonged with a gradual waning of effect so that, after a single dose, effective light sedation may continue throughout a lengthy appointment.

DISADVANTAGES

There are negative aspects to oral administration and, in selecting a treatment protocol for any given patient, these should be considered. One prime disadvantage is its dependence upon the cooperation of the patient. He must take the medication exactly as prescribed, following our instructions as to dose and time of administration. Many, while consciously aware of the value and need for these drugs, subconsciously resist. They tend to be forgetful and take the drugs improperly or not at all. Parents are often nervous about medicating their children and transmit these feelings to young patients, thereby raising obstacles in the path of effective treatment.

Adults, as a rule, ingest the drug in tablet or capsule form so that the size of the dose is accurate. Children, on the other hand, must often be given liquid preparations, which may be spilled and wasted should resistance be met during administration. Whether this results from simple uncooperativeness, fear, or objection to the taste of a given preparation does not alter the fact that children may not swallow the full dose, and suitable operating conditions will not be obtained.

For optimal results, medications must be taken at the proper time prior to the beginning of the treatment session to allow for absorption and onset of effect. Adequate sedation at the wrong time, or inadequate sedation at the right time, produces no benefit. When drugs are taken orally before the patient arrives at the office, we relinquish control over the time of administration. This difficulty can be countered by having the patient arrive early to take the medication on the premises and wait the onset time in the office.

Control of the ensuing level of sedation is poor, as there is great individual variation in response. The time required for onset of sedative effect after oral administration is sufficiently long to preclude the possibility of observing the result of a test dose and then altering the level as circumstances require. Dosages must be determined preoperatively, in a largely empirical manner.

Further difficulties are introduced because the established criteria for determining dosage for children on the basis of age or weight are unreliable for sedative medication. An extremely fearful child may require a disproportionate amount of drug when compared with the hypothetical average 150-pound adult. Sedation cannot be carried too deeply, since the level is related to external stimulation, and the child, after leaving the office and perceiving that the "danger" to him is past, may succumb to depression that causes him to sleep all day, much to the consternation of his parents. No amount of reassurance adequately comforts a parent whose child is still asleep six hours after returning home.

Control is sufficiently lacking so that deep sedation should not be attempted by this means. If a depression deeper than anticipated results, the level cannot be lightened and the patient may be put into a state of hynopsis, with the maintenance hazards of general anesthesia. When general anesthesia is used, it is done with inhalation or intravenous routes of administration which allow more positive control. Further, excessive sedation may produce sudden unexpected depression of the respiratory center or an abrupt fall in blood pressure, and in the usual treatment situation in which oral administration is used, the proper resuscitative capability would be lacking.

For lighter sedation, oral administration has its benefits and, when its limitations are recognized, it can be a valuable modality in dental practice.

AGENTS

Dosage and Reactions

Ideally, sedative medication should be effective after a single dose and many of our agents meet this requirement. Since the time of onset for most drugs is approximately one-half hour, the medication should be taken at least this far in advance of the beginning of treatment. With agents producing only a mild calming effect, the patient can be allowed to take the drug before arriving at the office. With drugs producing greater depression, administration should be accomplished in the office. For the patient's protection (and for your own), no one who has taken any sedative should be allowed to drive a car or operate machinery. Food in the stomach tends to retard absorption of many drugs, so patients usually do better if they have not eaten prior to the appointment.

Solid dosage forms (tablets, capsules) are preferable, since ingestion of the proper dosage is assured and there is no taste to which the patient may object. Just as patients may be unconsciously resistant to cooperating, they are similarly primed to dislike the taste of the preparation, no matter how pleasant *you* may think it is. It is awkward for us and unnecessarily expensive for the patient if a prescription is to be written for a single pill. If only one session will be required for treatment it is better to dispense the medication in the office; also, the patient cannot take an overdose.

In children attainment of proper dosage is complicated, since parents may not accurately measure the amount of liquid to be given. We think in terms of a standard apothecary teaspoon containing 5 ml. but household teaspoons vary greatly in capacity. Even though the child may swallow the full amount given to him, the measurement is subject to considerable variance.

If a liquid preparation is to be used it should be dispensed in a measured portion with the parents instructed to administer the full amount. We have found this procedure more reliable than prescribing the drug and relying upon the parents to measure a single dose. Further, it must be emphasized to the parents that the amount dispensed constitutes a single dose and must all be given at one time. Parents, in a naive attempt to be helpful or in fear of overdosing their child, often divide the dose and give it at intervals (possibly even some the night before); thus dooming the treatment session to failure. Further, it comforts parents in their desire to get full value for their money if they receive a full bottle of medicine. Try, if you can, to match the liquid volume to the size of the bottle and avoid dispensing partly filled bottles.

Even if the liquid is properly measured, there still remains the possibility that the child may cause some to be spilled from the spoon and receive an inadequate amount. To counter this difficulty we dispense a large disposable syringe (from which the needle has been removed) along with the medication. The parent is instructed to load the syringe with the liquid, introduce it into the child's mouth, and slowly squirt in the medication rather than offering it from a spoon. The child may still spit out some of the liquid but at least it gets in and that is half the battle. Results seem to be more reliable when liquids are given in this manner.

MANAGEMENT

Choice of drug and dosage determination depend upon several factors involving the needs of the patient, the properties of the drugs, and the requirements of the operative procedures. Sedation is not indicated only for the fearful patient who cannot accept dental treatment. Consider, also, the borderline patient who is intelligent enough to value the benefits of dental treatment and possesses adequate willpower and strength of character to stick it out but who, despite himself, fidgets, squirms, jerks his head, tenses his lip and cheek musculature and rinses incessantly. Some patients may be fine for short sessions but unable to tolerate long appointments (as for multiple crown preparations and impressions). Others may have no trouble accepting most procedures but may fear some specific one (surgery, root canal treatment, full mouth impressions). Many other indications come to mind: a transient but particularly trying personal situation (business or family troubles, menopause), reluctance to accept an analgesia mask, or nausea from deeper levels or prolonged contact with nitrous oxide. Finally, sedation is indicated for some patients because they request it.

Aside from the indication for sedation, we must also consider the depth required, availability of a responsible adult to accompany the patient home, time required for recovery, and how this will affect the patient's daily routine. Dosages cannot be expressed in absolute terms because patients, indications, and contraindications vary. The resultant effect can be altered by changing the drug as well as by modifying the dose. There is an acceptable range of dose for virtually every drug. Knowledge of previous reaction to a given drug will help in determining dose but this information is often unavailable. There is no substitute for professional judgment and, perhaps, a certain degree of intuition.

The following list of drugs classified according to use for adults, for both light (most common goal for oral administration) and more profound effects, and for children. In general, all should be taken about one-half hour before the beginning of treatment, because this represents the average latent period before onset of effect.

Adults

Patients in need of only slight relaxation will do well with chlordiazepoxide (Librium), diazepam (Valium), meprobamate (Equanil, Miltown) or ethinamate (Valmid). As a general rule they may be allowed to go home alone if they are dismissed about three hours after ingestion. However, drowsiness is possible and, if it occurs, driving should be prohibited, particularly with meprobamate.

Chlordiazepoxide may have optimal results only if the patient begins taking it a day or two before treatment with an extra dose one hour before. Ethinamate exhibits more rapid onset of effect than the others so this may be the drug of choice for administration in the office should the need for some mild sedation become evident at the time of treatment.

ADULTS

LIGHT EFFECT
Chlordiazepoxide (Librium)—10 mg. 3 times a day.
Diazepam (Valium)—2-5 mg.
Meprobamate (Equanil, Miltown)—200-400 mg.
Ethinamate (Valmid)—500 mg.

MODERATE EFFECT
Hydroxyzine (Atarax, Vistaril)—50-100 mg.
Promethazine (Phenergan)—50-100 mg.

MORE PROFOUND EFFECT
Secobarbital (Seconal)—100 mg.

The sedative effect of this first group of drugs is very mild and, in the absence of drowsiness, the patient is often unaware of any change but will remain more placid and calm when presented with a stressful situation. Concomitant use of analgesia is beneficial, but not mandatory, and its management is basically unchanged. As with all adjunctive sedation, less nitrous oxide can often be used and its administration terminated sooner.

Somewhat more pronounced (yet still light) sedation can be obtained through the use of either promethazine (Phenergan) or hydroxyzine (Atarax, Vistaril) in a dosage range of from 50 to 100 mg. Hydroxyzine is the more likely of the two drugs to produce drowsiness, while promethazine results in more of a dizzy, flying sensation. The patient appears quite relaxed and tends to close his eyes and appear asleep, but any sound or touch rouses him and he is quite able to carry on a lucid conversation. He will be able to get up and walk at any time. Promethazine, a phenothiazine derivative, will, in rare cases, produce deleterious extrapyramidal side effects that render treatment impossible. Hydroxyzine lacks this potential.

Still more profound sedation can be achieved with ingestion of secobarbital (Seconal) but, it must be remembered, since control is lacking, no attempt should be made to produce truly deep sedation. A grain and a half of secobarbital would probably be a sleep dose for the average patient if taken at home but, with the psychic stimulation of impending dental treatment, the effect is less profound. Patients will drowse but respond to stimuli. They will probably not be able to stand or ambulate unassisted for a couple of hours after onset of effect. Concomitant use of analgesia provides some additional depth and allows some "fine tuning" of the sedative effect, but this combination is for only the more experienced operators since the additive depression of both types of sedation may be sufficient to produce general anesthesia in some cases.

The patient will, undoubtedly, have to remain in the office for at least two hours after onset (and possibly longer). He will be able to walk out but will require some assistance. After arriving at home he should go to bed where he will probably sleep for a few hours. Family members should be instructed to allow the patient to sleep as long as he wishes and not to be concerned if this involves a good part of the day. Longer acting barbiturates should be avoided, as their recovery time is even more lengthy.

If the depression produced in this manner with secobarbital is inadequate, other means of sedation should be considered. Oral administration, in general, should be used only for lighter sedation and is not to be employed for deeper depression.

Children

As mentioned previously, liquid preparations are usually more practical for administration to child patients. Since barbiturates produce a paradoxic stimulating effect in some children their reliability is lessened. We have found chloral hydrate (Noctec) to be almost universally effective in a dose of 15 grains (10 ml. of syrup Noctec). An occasional tendency to gastric upset is countered by addition of 25 mg. of promethazine (5 ml. of Phenergan Fortis) to make a total of 1 tablespoon of liquid.

The two dosage forms, both syrups, are compatible. They will separate into two layers after standing, so the parents should be instructed to shake the bottle before administration. The optimal time for ingestion, as with virtually all oral sedatives, is about one-half hour before treatment. The classic rules for computing pediatric dosage on the basis of weight or age lack validity for sedative medication. Younger children (weighing less) usually require relatively more sedation so that the standard dose still applies to them even though they get more drug per pound of body weight. For very small children (weighing 35 pounds or less), though, it is usually better to halve the chloral hydrate (to 7½ grains).

The effect is variable. Some children will appear to be asleep in the reception room while others will be only somewhat dizzy and ataxic. In the dental chair, most come to life but a few resist placement of an analgesia mask. Management is almost universally successful when combined with analgesia. Whatever the result in the chair, the vast majority of these children sleep for several hours after they return home.

13 | Intramuscular Administration

Injection into a muscle forms a reservoir of medication that is gradually absorbed into the circulating blood. Properly given, intra-muscular injection represents one of the safest means of drug administration, producing few complications and achieving more reliable sedation than after medication by mouth.

ADVANTAGES AND DISADVANTAGES

The need for patient cooperation is reduced because agents can be given in the office at the optimal time and in controlled doses. Drugs can be effective in a single dose without the need for several day's management, as is sometimes the case with oral administration. There is more latitude in drug selection, since gastric irritation or destruction of the compound by digestive juices is not a factor. Absorption, in general, is more reliable than with oral administration, resulting in a latent period (until onset of effect) which is more standard and predictable.

An anesthetic mask, which might be objectionable or frightening to some patients need not be used. Premedication by injection may aid a previously resistant patient to accept analgesia. Few persons, even those who will not tolerate an intraoral injection, will object to one in the arm. Acceptance of analgesia and its concomitant use often paves the way for acceptance of the injection by those few who fear it.

There is neither taste nor odor to bother the patient. The procedure is over quickly and should be well tolerated. A choice of sites is available. With the use of disposable needles and adherence to certain basic precepts, pain is minimal. Aseptic technique is essential, and if scrupulously followed, complications at the injection site are rare.

The dentist is required to stock some drugs and use special armamentarium but this presents no real problem. Disposable syringes, supplied in sterile packaging, are extremely inexpensive. The armamentarium and preparation are considerably simpler than those required for intravenous administration. No preparation other than opening a package and loading a syringe is necessary. Certain agents are supplied already loaded in disposable syringes or in carpule form for special syringes. The number of drugs to be inventoried can be kept small, their cost is slight, and they can be stored for some time.

Some specialized knowledge and dexterity are needed in making the injections but, compared with the vast range of expertise and skill required to practice dentistry, this poses no major problem. With careful attention to detail and some familiarity with anatomy and landmarks, any dentist is capable of making the injections. No really new technique must be mastered, since we are all experienced in the intramuscular injection of local anesthetics in the mouth. With only a slight change in armamentarium and orientation the procedure is basically the same.

Time required until onset of effect is predictable but is sufficiently prolonged to preclude alteration of dose on the

114

basis of observed response. As with oral administration, dosage must be determined, somewhat empirically, in advance. We cannot give a test dose and alter the effect produced, since further injection would require too long a waiting period to be practical. Similarly, we cannot lighten the ensuing level, as is possible with inhalation agents. In view of these circumstances, sedation should be kept relatively light since depth would be obtained without control and this would be a potentially dangerous situation and one to be avoided. Also, since the sedation produced is fairly prolonged, the recovery time might be too protracted for our ambulatory type of office management in which the patient must be discharged, in the care of laymen, to return home. With poorly accessible veins, however, this remains a prime method of choice for sedative medication.

TECHNIQUE OF INJECTION

For proper effect and avoidance of complications, injections must be made with attention to detail rather than carelessly or mechanically. To avoid puncturing major nerves or blood vessels, you must know the anatomy of the various injection sites. The entire area must be fully exposed to provide an unobstructed view. The needle must be long enough to deposit the solution well within the selected muscle mass which should be relaxed and large enough to accommodate the volume of solution to be injected. Only relatively small quantities are given intramuscularly. Drugs should be injected slowly in order to allow the muscle to distend and prevent their escape into surrounding tissues. The site must be sufficiently immobilized to allow careful technique, producing minimal irritation and discomfort with maximal safety and reliability.

Always aspirate the syringe before injecting to prevent accidental intravascular injection. While the agents may be compatible with intravenous administration, the management is quite different and not to be stumbled into inadvertently. Appearance of blood in the syringe upon aspirating necessitates movement of the needle tip in the tissues before injecting. Never inject while inserting the needle because aspiration cannot be performed at this time and also because tracking of the drug in the superficial tissues predisposes to a greater likelihood of irritation. Many solutions are inherently irritating and should be deposited only well within a muscle mass.

Sterile technique must be scrupulously followed. Use only uncontaminated disposable syringes, needles and medications. Drug vials or ampules must be carefully protected from contamination. Complications at the injection site can almost invariably be attributed to faulty injection technique or lack of asepsis.

Injection Sequence

Before injection, clean the skin at the site and approximately two inches around it with a sponge wet with a suitable solution such as alcohol. If you are right-handed (if left-handed, reverse all directions) then grasp muscle and skin between the thumb and index finger of the left hand, pinching tissue to produce some surface anesthesia and raising the muscle away from deeper soft tissue structures and bone. In general, the left hand immobilizes the tissue and syringe and the right hand injects.

Holding the barrel of the syringe perpendicular to the skin in a dart grip, quickly thrust the needle through the surface of the skin and then, firmly and steadily, carry it deeper until about

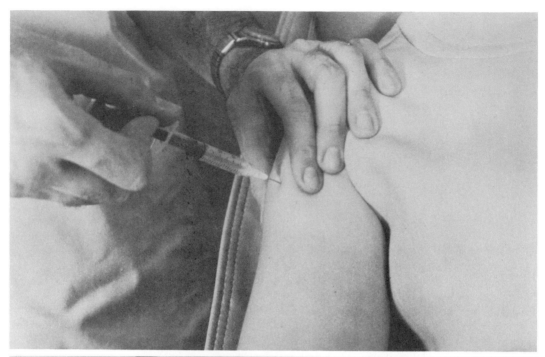

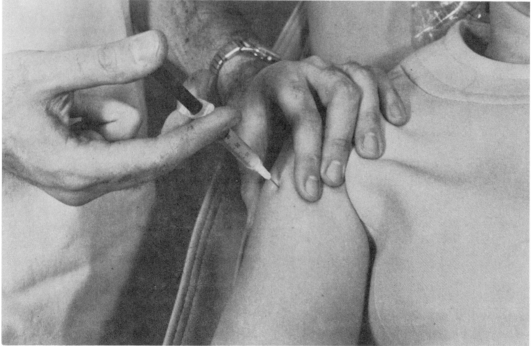

FIG. 29. While immobilizing the tissue and supporting the syringe perpendicular to the surface of the skin (A) exert a negative back pressure on the plunger to test for positive aspiration. After establishing that no blood appears, (B) slowly and steadily press in the plunger with the thumb while gripping the side extensions of the barrel with the index and middle fingers.

three-fourths of its length is buried. Most of the pain associated with injection is felt during the skin puncture, so this is completed quickly. Leaving some of the needle exposed provides a means of removal should breakage occur.

When the desired depth is attained, transfer the syringe to the left hand and with the right hand exert a negative back pressure on the plunger to test for positive aspiration. If any blood appears in the syringe partially withdraw it and readvance slightly to the side or insert at another site. If no blood appears, with the right thumb slowly and steadily press in the plunger as far as it will go, while the index and midde fingers grip the side extensions of the barrel. Never inject unless aspiration is negative. Always inject slowly.

The needle is withdrawn while pressure is exerted on the site with an alcohol sponge applied in order to reduce the possibility of leakage of medication into the subcutaneous tissues, thereby lessening the risk of irritation. Massaging the area will enhance and accelerate absorption. With an alcohol sponge clean any blood or agent leaking from the skin puncture and cover the area with an adhesive bandage to prevent staining of clothing. The patient can be instructed to remove the bandage a short time later.

Do not trust to memory. Make an immediate record of the name and amount of agent, time of injection, method of administration and any pertinent observations relative to patient reaction.

Injection Sites

Generally speaking, injection can be made at any site that meets the criteria of ease of access, adequate visibility, size of muscle mass, safe distance from major nerves and vessels, and shallowness of subcutaneous fatty layer.

Mid-deltoid Area

Because of its ease of access the mid-deltoid area is most commonly used for intramuscular injections. The muscle mass is smaller than that of the gluteal area so it will not tolerate repeated injections or deposition of large amounts of solution. The effect upon the patient's sense of modesty is, however, less.

With the patient sitting, the entire prominence of the deltoid in the upper arm should be exposed. A man can remove his shirt if the sleeve cannot be rolled up that high. If a woman cannot expose the area, she can remove one arm from her blouse and cover herself before you enter the room to perform the injection, or she can be given a short-sleeved smock to change into. Keeping such a smock in the office saves the day many a time.

The muscle represents quite a pronounced mass on the lateral side of the upper arm below the shoulder prominence. Avoiding the acromion, clavicle and humerus, injection is made into the middle of the muscle mass. Some operators believe that the patient will experience less soreness later if injection is made at the same height but more posteriorly into the posterior triceps, a muscle that moves less during arm function. In any event, do not go too low as this can be dangerously close to the radial nerve.

Gluteal Area

Requiring some disrobing, the gluteal area, while actually a better injection site, is rarely used in adults. For obstreperous children, though, it offers the advantage of ease of immobilization. The child's movements can be controlled during injection while he is held across the lap of the parent in the classic spanking position.

The gluteal area and buttocks are not synonymous. The buttocks, composed mainly of fatty tissue, are situated inferiorly to the gluteal musculature. To avoid the sciatic nerve and superior gluteal artery, injections should be made into the upper outer quadrant of the gluteal area. This places the injection site closer to the iliac crest than to the prominence of the buttocks.

Ideally, the patient should be lying face down with the feet toed in to relax the muscles. The needle is inserted perpendicularly to the surface upon which the patient is lying and directed straight down. Since the muscle mass is greatest here, this site carries with it the greatest tolerance to bulk of solution and irritating properties of drugs.

Anterior Thigh

Another available site, perhaps not too often used, is the vastus lateralis area on the anterior (ventral) aspect of

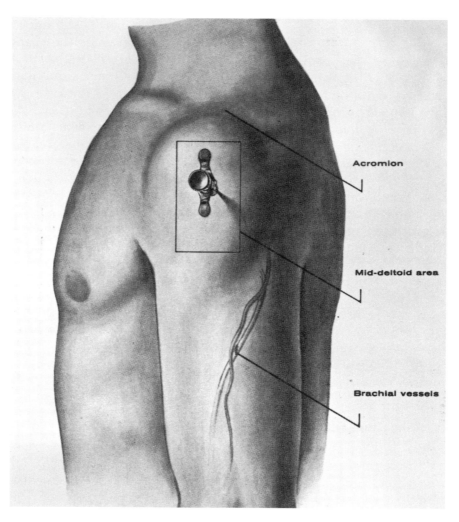

Acromion

Mid-deltoid area

Brachial vessels

Fig. 30. The mid-deltoid site for intramuscular injection. (Courtesy Wyeth Laboratories, Philadelphia, Pa.)

the thigh. This site is sufficiently removed from major nerves and vessels,
providing both a shallow subcutaneous
fatty layer and adequate muscle den-
sity. Adequate exposure can be obtained with the patient sitting or lying
on his back. This is basically the area
that would show between the top of a
woman's stocking and the bottom of
her girdle. With minimal clothing de-
rangement and loss of modesty, she
could expose the area by raising the
hem of her skirt.

ARMAMENTARIUM

Transmission of infectious disease
(including hepatitis) is minimized by
use of disposable syringes and needles.
They also require the least effort in
preparation and enhance patient tolerance because their sharpness minimizes
pain. The sharpness of the needle is
more important in avoiding discomfort
than is its gauge. Use of sterile dis-
posal injection supplies is virtually
mandatory today in light of prevailing

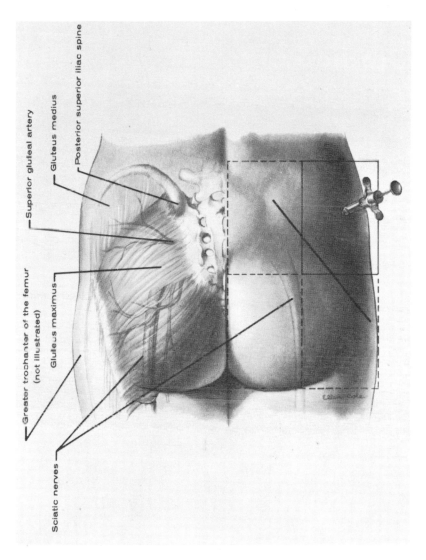

FIG. 31. The gluteal site for intramuscular injection. (Courtesy
Wyeth Laboratories, Philadelphia, Pa.)

standards of practice considered in professional negligence suits.

For most injections a 3 or 5 ml. syringe is adequate, and this should be fitted with a 22-gauge needle 1½ inches in length. The only other supplies needed are a sponge (2″ x 2″) wet with alcohol, an adhesive bandage and the drugs to be injected.

Many agents are supplied by the manufacturers in sterile, airtight, rubber-sealed multiple-dose vials. With these vials, remove the safety seal and dust cap and cleanse the stopper with alcohol. Inject into the vial a volume of air equal to the amount of solution to be removed then hold upside down so that the needle tip is below the level of the solution and withdraw the plunger to aspirate the desired amount of solution. Leave the needle in the vial until time for the injection. The vial

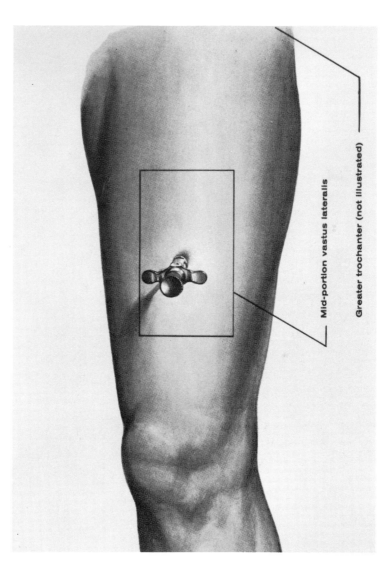

Fig. 32. The anterior thigh site for intramuscular injection. (Courtesy Wyeth Laboratories, Philadelphia, Pa.)

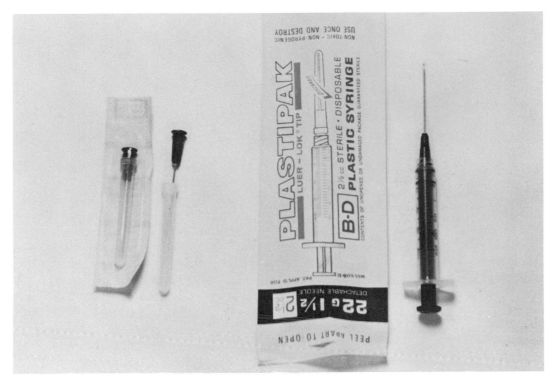

Fig. 33. Disposable needle and syringe as supplied in sterile packaging.

serves as a sterile, labelled cover for the needle. If the syringe is to be removed from the vial while awaiting use, it should be labelled after recovering the needle with the same cover with which it was supplied. Again cleanse the stopper on the vial and cover for storage.

Some agents are supplied in unit dosage in sealed glass ampules. These are made with a constricted neck intended to be broken at a scored line. Grasping both ends of the ampule, bend it until it breaks. Always protect your hands against shattering of the glass by holding the ampule wrapped in a towel or other cloth. The broken ampule is not airtight, so no air need be injected prior to removal of the solution. It is necessary only to insert the needle (without contamination by touching the outside or the sides of the open neck), holding the ampule upright and aspirating the agent into the syringe. Hold the syringe with the needle up and expel any air bubble it may contain, label the syringe, and cap the needle until use.

MANAGEMENT

The latent period between intramuscular injection of sedative medication and onset of effect usually lasts about 20 minutes. Treatment can be efficiently begun after a half hour has elapsed. The duration is on the order of two to three hours from onset with an early peak and then a gradual decline. Sedative depth wanes as time progresses but the patient, being awake and experiencing no pain, usually accepts the procedure. Thus the waning of sedative effect is paralleled by a de-

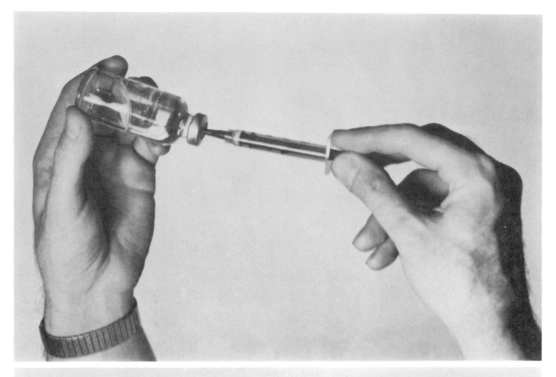

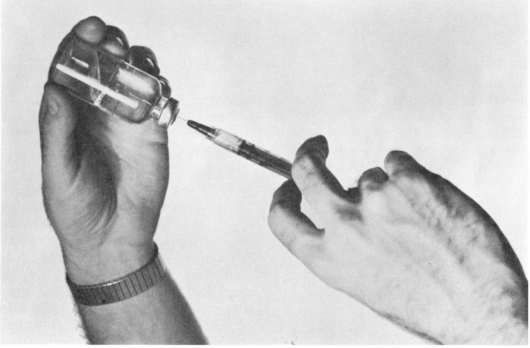

Fig. 34. When removing solution from a multiple dose vial, (A) first inject into the vial a volume of air equal to the amount of solution to be removed and then (B) with the needle tip below the level of the solution, withdraw the plunger to aspirate the desired amount of solution.

creased need for it. In effect, the recovery period begins during treatment if only the single original dose is given (Fig. 37). Patients can almost always leave the office (accompanied by a responsible adult) within an hour after a 1½-hour appointment. They often remain somewhat sedated for a good part of the appointment day and should rest at home. They should not drive a car for the remainder of the day.

Control is achieved by virtue of the elimination of the need for patient cooperation. The time of administration and size of dose are accurately known. The dosage, as with oral administration, must be predetermined somewhat empirically, since the latent period is sufficiently long to preclude injection

of additional amounts after the effects of the first dose are seen.

The patient is seated and the injection given at the selected site. One half hour is allowed to elapse while the patient remains comfortably seated in the dental chair. The surroundings should be quiet and there should be no traffic through the room. The less the patient is stimulated, the greater the sedative effect. Analgesia can be used during the injection, then stopped for the waiting period, and resumed during treatment. As the case progresses, the analgesia can often be reduced or stopped while the mask is left in place and the patient is given oxygen to breathe (or the inhaling valve can be opened for access to room air). Total cessation of

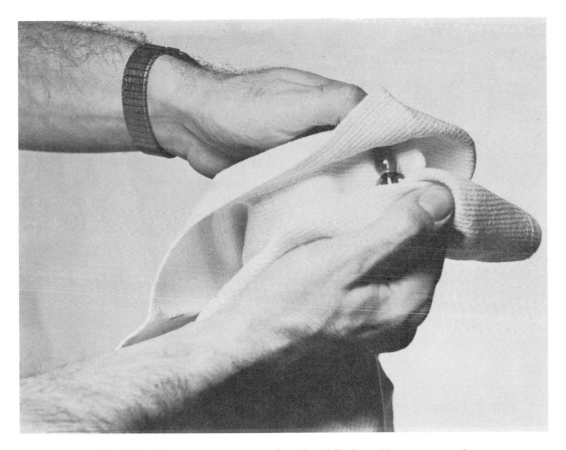

FIG. 35. Always protect your hands while breaking an ampule.

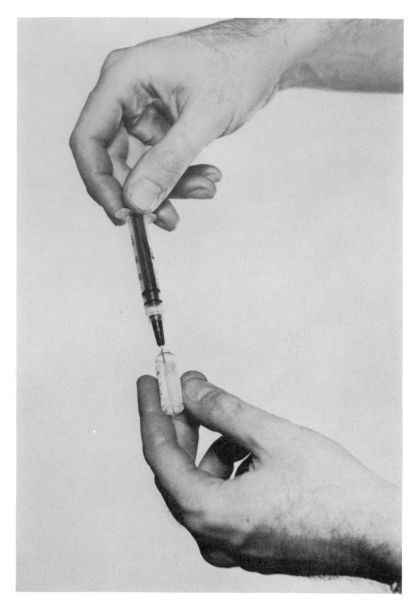

FIG. 36. The broken ampule is not airtight so no air need be injected prior to removal of solution but aseptic technique is still essential.

gas flow with a closed inhaling valve can cause a sensation of suffocation and must always be avoided.

Because of the more reliable absorption after intramuscular injection, the ensuing sedation is not as subject to the wide variations of effect seen with oral administration. Deeper sedation should not be attempted orally because an inadvertently profound result can produce sedation that is dangerously deep. Dosages must be calculated so as to keep the patient lightly sedated. With intramuscular injection we can safely strive for somewhat greater depth than with oral administration

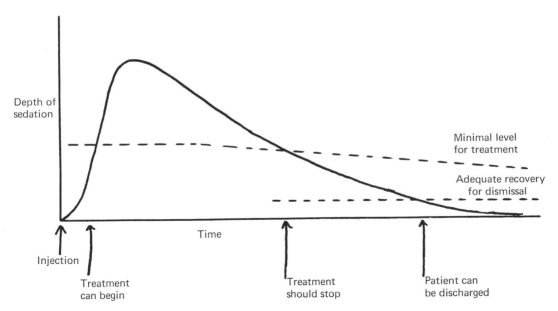

FIG. 37. Sedative effect following a single intramuscular injection. After a latent period there is relatively rapid attainment of peak activity and then a gradual waning of effect.

since, with the greater reliability, variation is lessened. Relatively greater doses can be given. For extremely light levels, the simplicity of oral administration is preferable.

AGENTS

Dosages and Reactions

Chlordiazepoxide (Librium) in a dose of 50 to 100 mg. may leave the patient feeling unchanged or may provoke very slight drowsiness. The ability to withstand stress better will certainly be apparent to the doctor if not to the patient. Diazepam (Valium) is more likely to produce some drowsiness and lethargy but its effect is still mild. Amnesia is variable and certainly not as pronounced as with its administration intravenously. Patients receiving promethazine (Phenergan) or hydroxyzine (Atarax, Vistaril) often appear to be asleep but will react readily to the spoken word or to operative manipulation. Both drugs are markedly anti-

emetic so they complement analgesia quite well not only by lessening the concentration of nitrous oxide needed (and the duration of its administration) but also by countering its nauseating properties.

MODERATE EFFECT
  Chlordiazepoxide (Librium) — 50-100 mg.
  Diazepam (Valium)—5-10 mg.
  Promethazine (Phenergan)—50-100 mg.
  Hydroxyzine (Atarax, Vistaril)—50-100 mg.
MORE PROFOUND EFFECT
  Secobarbital (Seconal)—50-100 mg.
  { Secobarbital (Seconal)—50-100 mg.
  { Promethazine (Phenergan)—25 mg.
  { Promethazine (Phenergan)—50 mg.
  { Meperidine (Demerol)—50-100 mg.

Secobarbital (Seconal), given in a dose of 100 mg. intramuscularly, would probably constitute an hypnotic dose for many patients if they were not subjected to the stimulation of dental treatment. The high alkalinity of the solution renders it quite irritating, so care must be exerted to inject well within the muscle mass. The solution (as with all irritating drugs) should not be injected until the needle reaches its full depth. Tracking the solution through the subcutaneous tissues predisposes to postoperative soreness at the injection site.

If 100 mg. of secobarbital does not produce adequate sedation it would be better to combine it with another agent rather than to increase its dosage. Safety is maintained by not heavily loading the cerebral tissues with large amounts of the one drug. Promethazine (25 mg.) serves as an effective synergist for the secobarbital (reduced to 75 mg.) but the two solutions are incompatible and must be injected from separate syringes, preferably at different sites (e.g., both arms). No solution that becomes cloudy or forms a precipitate should ever be injected. If the phenothiazine derivative, promethazine, must be avoided for a given patient, a combination of secobarbital and a similar dose of hydroxyzine can be substituted. If the patient is too lightly sedated to remain cooperative, the dose of secobarbital can be increased to 100 mg. at subsequent sessions. With repeated trials the ideal dose can be established for each patient.

An alternate drug combination for fairly profound sedation is 75 mg. of meperidine (Demerol) with 25 mg. of promethazine. This combination is very often used for operating room presurgical sedation. The drugs are compatible and may be combined in a single syringe. However, to minimize injection site soreness, the smallest volume possible should be injected. Meperidine can be obtained in a 100 mg. per ml. strength (50 mg. per ml. is also available) for reduction of the volume necessary but extreme care is required in measuring it. The more concentrated the solution the easier it is to err in measuring and the more care is required. If the dosage is to be varied at further sessions, the meperidine is the one to change. The acceptable range is 50 to 100 mg.

It must be remembered that the greater the sedation, the greater the depression of vital centers. If deeper sedation is to be employed, vital signs must be carefully monitored. Respiratory function, particularly, tends to be depressed. Adequate means and skill for its maintenance must be available.

This technique is one of sedation and not anesthesia. All of the drug combinations described must be supplemented with local anesthesia. While it is possible to treat some patients without local anesthesia, sedated patients should always be pain-free if the method is to be successful. Experience of pain will wreck any sedative regimen.

Concomitant use of nitrous oxide analgesia is not mandatory but almost always improves the management. The additional sedation derived from the nitrous oxide necessitates modification of the injected dosage since the two are additive. Even if no nitrous oxide is given, the movements of the breathing bag provide an effective means of monitoring respiratory function. In the cases where analgesia is not used but a breathing bag is desired, straight oxygen should be given so that the patient does not experience interference with inspiration.

14 | Intravenous Administration

Introduction of sedative drugs into a vein eliminates the delay encountered upon waiting for absorption into the bloodstream and produces an almost instantaneous blood level, so individual reaction can be immediately visualized and control is enhanced. If safety is to be considered a function of controllability, then intravenous administration, carefully employed, is extremely safe and approaches inhalation in this respect.

ADVANTAGES AND DISADVANTAGES

Onset of effect is extremely rapid. The arm-brain circulation time is only about 25 sec., so that after only this short period the agents begin to exert their effect on brain tissue. Delivery to the brain occurs so rapidly that injection must be made slowly to avoid a precipitous cerebral effect that could push the patient past our desired levels of sedation.

Predetermined amounts need not be given empirically because a small test dose can be injected, the effect observed and adjustment made to deepen the level. When dilute solutions are injected slowly, the patient can be titrated to a fairly precise level of depression and maintained in that state. Unlike most inhalation agents (except Trilene) intravenous drugs must be chemically degraded by the body and the metabolites excreted so the blood level and depressive state cannot be altered at will. Overdosage, which can result in dangerous depression or production of a general anesthetic state, can be avoided by careful, slow injection of small amounts per unit time to bring the patient gradually to the desired level. Because of the degree of control possible, sedation can be carried deeper than with oral or intramuscular administration. Recovery time, while longer than that usually seen following inhalation, is notably shorter than that obtained after administration by these other routes.

An additional safety factor inherent in intravenous administration is the availability of an avenue for introduction of emergency or supportive drugs should their use become necessary. All drugs, when introduced into the venous system, exert their effect more rapidly than when given by other routes and the emergency drugs are no different. Also, the corrective effect of these drugs is more predictable and, since their action can be immediately observed, corrective increments need be added only as needed.

The potential for rapid increase in the level of depression and fairly speedy withdrawal of agent from the circulating blood to lighten the level as the case progresses necessitates a close watch of depth and constant monitoring of vital signs. Since patients undergoing sedative management remain within the first stage of anesthesia (analgesia), the classic Guedel signs are not valid parameters for gauging depth, since they will not be seen. Frequently, additional doses must be added during prolonged management, but the attention required is not so great as to distract the experienced practitioner from his operative procedures.

127

Venipuncture technique represents a a special skill that must be mastered through practice. Dentists as a rule exhibit a high degree of manual dexterity that should allow them to attain this capability with relative ease in a short time. Patients at first should be carefully selected on the basis of suitability of superficial veins. In obese persons the veins are usually difficult to locate and aged patients often present fragile or sclerotic vessels that militate against successful management. Venipuncture for uncooperative children can be impossible. In any case, it is unwise to persist in attempts at venipuncture in the face of failure. At this point the patient is unsedated, and exposure to painful multiple needle punctures may create a state of anxiety which cannot effectively be overcome with sedative management. It is wiser, in this eventuality, to abandon intravenous administration for the time being and to rely instead on inhalation with or without intramuscular injection of drugs.

Vein walls lack pain sensation and the major cause of discomfort is the skin puncture. Once the needle has been advanced into the vein and fixed to the skin there should be no further discomfort to the patient. Irritating solutions, if they remain in the area too long, may produce some awareness of discomfort in the arm proximal to the injection site. Care must be given to allow unimpeded flow of solutions in the vein by not strapping the arm to the armboard too tightly, by assuring proper needle position and by maintaining adequate flow of solution in the infusion. Use of nitrous oxide analgesia at the time of venipuncture usually eliminates even the slight discomfort that may be involved.

Some local complications are possible at the venipuncture site both during and after management but, with careful aseptic technique they are infrequent and amenable to treatment. A more complete discussion can be found in Chapter 15.

Respiratory depression is a constant possibility with deep intravenous sedation because of direct effect on higher centers and because of the lack of excitation of respiratory tract reflexes as often seen with use of general anesthetic gases.

CONTRAINDICATIONS

Intravenous administration is contraindicated in the absence of palpable visible superficial veins or if there is inadequate function of detoxifying organs (most often the liver). A preoperative airway problem and failure of the patient to arrange for the presence of a responsible adult to accompany him home also are causes for cancelling the case. No patient, no matter how alert he may seem, should ever be allowed to drive a car or leave the office unaccompanied. With a patient maintained in the analgesia stage, aspiration of matter into the tracheobronchial tree is not a likely occurrence. However, there is the possibility that he may inadvertently enter the general anesthetic state. Vomitus can severely hamper treatment so all patients could be required to maintain an empty stomach prior to treatment. Failure to meet this requirement should result in postponement of the case.

TECHNIQUE
OF VENIPUNCTURE

Venipuncture, properly performed, should cause almost no pain and should be virtually free of complications or uncomfortable sequelae. Care must be taken to assure that nerves and arteries are avoided and that all supplies and equipment are uncontaminated. Any vein can serve as a portal for entry of medication. To facilitate needle place-

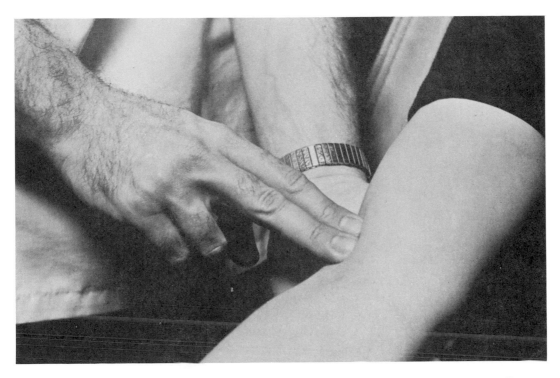

FIG. 38. Before applying the tourniquet, palpate the selected vessel to confirm the lack of arterial pulsations.

ment, evaluate all veins and choose the largest, straightest, most accessible one. The vein must be clearly visible. Never probe blindly for a vein. With the arm in a relaxed position, and before applying the tourniquet, the vessel selected should be palpated and demonstrated to be free of arterial pulsations.

The arm must be firmly supported and controlled to avoid movement during puncture, and the overlying tissues as well as the vein must be fixed. The delicacy of movement and fine control that are required would be impossible on a moving target. Further, the operator himself should maintain a comfortable posture, not unbalanced or awkward, so that he can maintain control.

Never inject unless aspiration has produced a positive show of dark venous blood. Always inject slowly. It is easier to control the dosages injected and to maintain a slow rate if the solutions are dilute.

Concomitant use of nitrous oxide analgesia overcomes the slight discomfort of venipuncture for most patients. Spraying the puncture site with ethyl chloride or raising a skin wheal with approximately 0.5 ml. of local anesthetic solution are alternate methods.

With practice, the entire procedure can be completed quickly and painlessly. Prepare all materials, keep them closely at hand and use inconspicuously and without unnecessary delays to avoid compounding any fear or anxiety.

Injection Sequence

Prepare all supplies before ushering the patient into the treatment room. If the needle is to be attached to a syringe during venipuncture, test the syringe to see that it is working properly and that

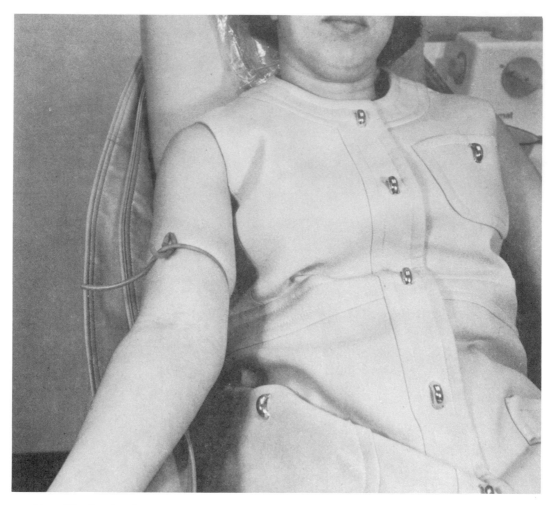

FIG. 39. Apply the tourniquet with a slipknot and place a few inches proximal to the venipuncture site.

the needle is patent. If the needle is on an infusion set, bleed all air out of the tubing by allowing the solution to run through it. Inspect the needle point (without touching it) to be certain that it is properly ground and without burs.

With the patient's arm in a position that is relaxed for him and at a comfortable working height for you, look for suitable veins. Take your time. Examine all the possible areas on both forearms and hands. Application of a tourniquet a few inches proximal to the bend of the elbow distends the veins and makes them more visible. Apply the

tourniquet tightly without pinching skin or pulling hair. Ideally, enough occlusive pressure should be applied to obstruct venous outflow without stopping arterial inflow to the arm. Presence of arterial pulsation should be tested for only before tourniquet placement.

Allow time for venous filling. Distension of the veins is aided if the patient repeatedly closes and opens his fist (later keeping it clenched while the needle is inserted). Some slight venous spasm may prevent filling and distension. This can be countered by lightly

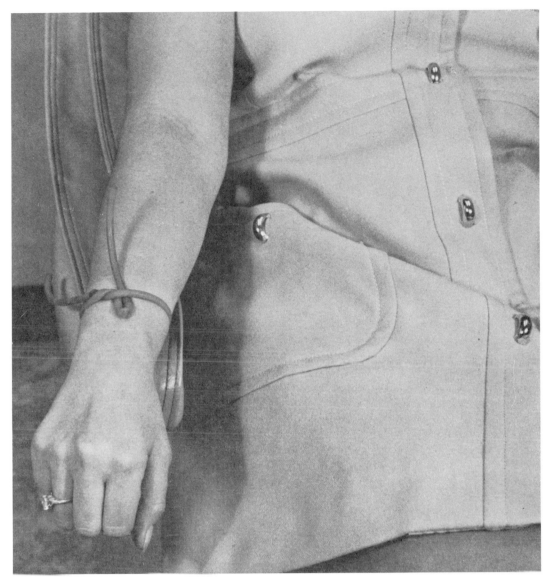

Fig. 40. For venipuncture on the hand, place the tourniquet just proximal to the wrist joint.

slapping the projected puncture site or flicking it with a finger. If there is still no vein that stands out enough to be considered suitable, remove the tourniquet, let the arm hang down for a few minutes, then reapply the tourniquet and try again. Venous spasm resulting from an adrenergic reaction to anxiety often can be overcome by premedicating the patient on another day or by use of nitrous oxide analgesia. If one arm provides no suitable vein, try the other one. There is no place in this technique for heroics. If no vein is suitable for venipuncture, chose another method of sedation.

Always place the tourniquet a few inches proximal to the anticipated puncture site. If venipuncture is to be attempted on the hand or at the wrist,

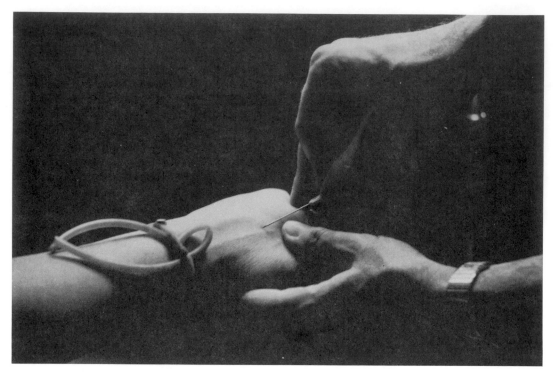

FIG. 41. With the bevel up and the needle at a 30-degree angle to the skin and parallel to the long axis of the vein but just to its side, aim the needle point to make its skin penetration about one-quarter inch below the point where you plan to enter the vein.

move the tourniquet down from the upper arm.

Once the vein and site of injection have been selected, cleanse the area with alcohol. Grip the arm with left hand (for a right-handed operator) and with the thumb stretch the skin distally to immobilize the vein and facilitate puncturing. Be careful not to obstruct the path of injection with your thumb. With the bevel up, hold the needle at a 30-degree angle to the skin and parallel to the long axis of the vein but just to its side. Aim the needle point about one-quarter inch below the point where the needle will enter the vein and thrust through the skin. Flatten the needle angle so that it is almost flush with the skin, swing the tip sideways to the vein and, with the bevel still up, engage the vein wall and enter the vessel. If aspiration is positive, ad-

vance the needle further until at least two-thirds of its length lies within the lumen of the vein.

If a syringe is used, test aspiration by holding the needle hub with the left hand and pull back on the plunger with the right. If dark venous blood appears in the barrel, the tourniquet can be removed and the injection begun.

If the needle is attached directly to an infusion set, aspiration is tested by pinching and releasing the latex injection site, looking for a reflux of blood into the clear tubing near the needle adapter. If aspiration is positive, remove the tourniquet and open the clamp to test for free flow of the infusion. If flow is poor or absent, perhaps the needle lumen is covered by vein wall. Rotate the needle or withdraw it a few millimeters while watching the drip chamber for flow rate.

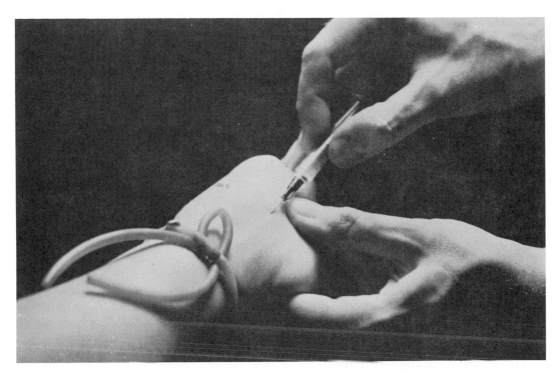

FIG. 42. While holding the skin taut with the thumb, insert the needle through the skin.

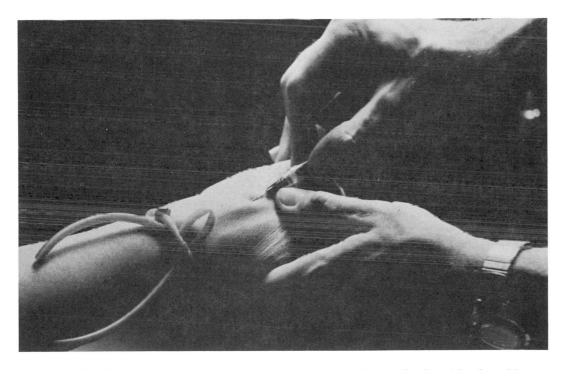

FIG. 43. Flatten the needle angle so that it is almost flush with the skin, swing the needle tip sideways to the vein and, with the bevel still up, engage the vein wall and enter the vessel.

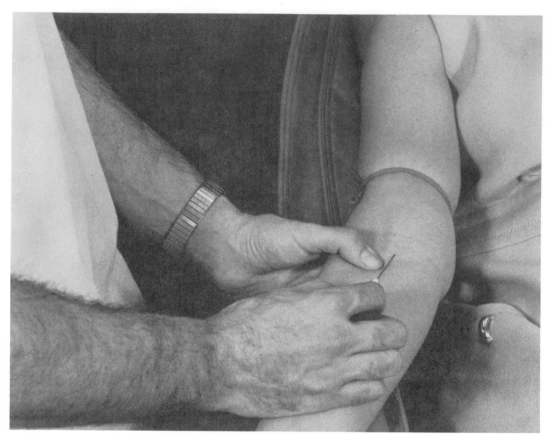

Fig. 44. The technique is the same at the elbow or any other site. While holding the skin taut, parallel the needle to the long axis of the vein and accomplish venipuncture in the same two-step procedure.

Never advance the needle when no tourniquet has been applied. Propping the needle hub away from the skin with a rolled gauze square (2″ x 2″) sometimes improves the flow. If flow is still too slow, try raising the bottle. If proper flow cannot be established or if a swelling forms around the puncture site (extravasation of fluid), withdraw the needle and try in another vein or proximally in the same vein (never distal to a previous puncture). When good flow is confirmed, place one piece of half-inch tape across the needle hub, then loop the tubing (form a circle of about 3 to 4 inches diameter) back to the puncture site and place a second piece of tape across the puncture and

the recurved tubing. Be careful that the tape does not obscure the clear tubing next to the needle so that aspiration can be checked later in the management. The needle can be left in place throughout the case and drugs injected whenever necessary.

Throughout this time, while the vein is entered and the needle fixed, the arm must have been held immobile to prevent movement or flexion of a joint that could have dislodged the needle. For the remainder of the case the arm can be held immobile by strapping to an armboard with one length of 1-in. wide tape proximal to the joint and one length distal. The board should be lightly padded for comfort yet firm

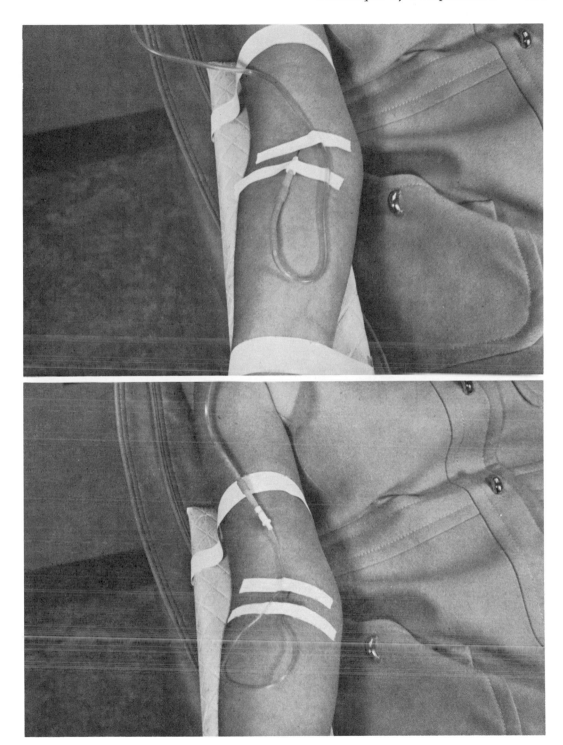

FIG. 45. Whether with (A) a needle with a conventional hub or (B) a butterfly needle, the fixation is the same. The first tape holds the needle and the second tape maintains the loop in the tubing and covers the puncture site.

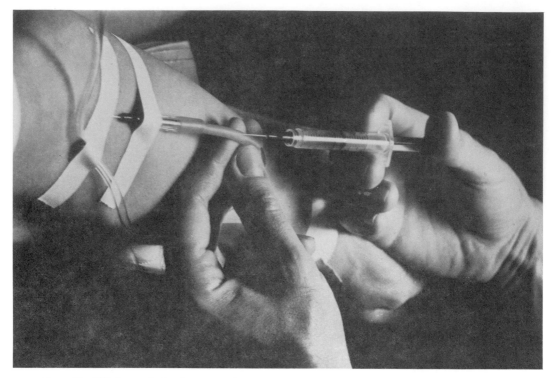

FIG. 46. With an infusion running, leave the needle in the vein throughout the case and make any further injection into the latex injection site in the infusion tubing.

enough to prevent joint movement. The taping should be tight enough for immobilization yet not so tight as to restrict venous return. With the arm positioned comfortably, the armboard should be taped to the chair arm.

When the needle is removed, care must be taken to prevent hemorrhage from the resultant hole in the vessel wall. While holding the needle hub, remove the tape and press over the puncture area with an alcohol sponge. Withdraw the needle, maintain the pressure for a minute or so and then cover with a tight adhesive bandage. The bandage will press tightly if one side is affixed to the skin and the bandage is pulled across the puncture site (tightly enough to crease the skin) before the other side is pressed firmly down. Always warn the patient that a hematoma may form in the area of the puncture and that it will fade in a few days as with any other black and blue mark.

Venipuncture Sites

Generally speaking, venipuncture usually can be performed in any sufficiently large and accessible vein but, for practicality, we limit our choice to those of the antecubital fossa at the elbow, the forearm and the dorsum of the hand.

The antecubital fossa usually contains the largest superficial veins in the arm. They are quite close to the surface and, being well supported in subcutaneous tissue, do not roll, thus facilitating needle entry. Unfortunately, the brachial artery which also traverses this area, is quite large and variable, dividing into the ulnar and radial arteries sometimes proximally to the

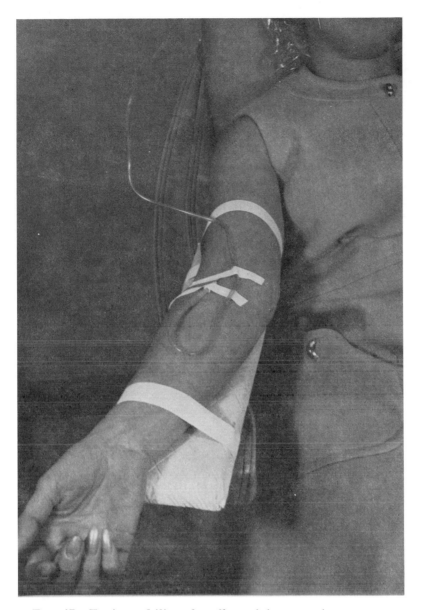

FIG. 47. To immobilize the elbow joint tape it to an arm board with one tape proximal and one tape distal to the joint.

bend of the elbow and sometimes distally. Always palpate carefully for arterial pulsation before applying the tourniquet as this artery can be rather superficial in some patients and be mistaken for a vein.

The dorsal digital plexus of veins on the hand presents a greater incidence of anatomic variation but this is of lesser concern, since the arteries in the area are smaller and deeper, thereby notably reducing the danger of inadvertent entry. The individual veins tend to be more tortuous and poorly supported in the subcutaneous tissues than those at the elbow. Any vein selected must have a straight segment at least as long as the length of needle to be

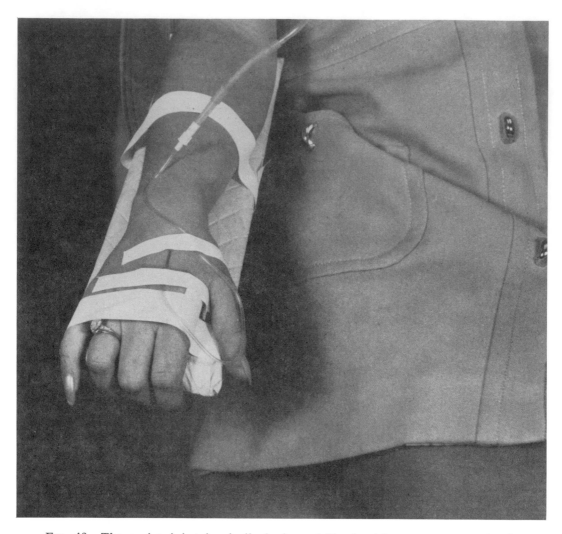

Fig. 48. The wrist joint is similarly immobilized with one tape proximal to the wrist joint and one tape distal (covering the four fingers but not the thumb).

inserted. Extra care must be exerted to fix the skin and immobilize rolling veins during needle insertion. The veins here, being small, have thin walls that are easily ruptured and tend to leak fluids during infusion or blood after needle withdrawal. Hematoma formation, while possible after cessation of the infusion at any site, is more common here, so pressure must be applied for a longer time after removal of the needle.

Venipuncture at the antecubital fossa requires armboard immobilization of the elbow throughout the management and this may prove quite uncomfortable for many. Fixation of the wrist, as is necessary with venipuncture on the hand, does not cause as much discomfort because most of the arm can be left relatively free to move. Needle insertion within the forearm, away from all joints, does not require any arm fixation (other than preventing the arm from falling) since no flexion is possible in this area. This can be the most comfortable of all sites.

In general, we insert the smallest needle allowing adequate flow into the largest, most convenient vein. Veins

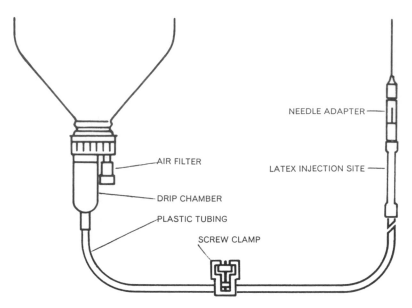

FIG. 49. Diagram representing the parts of an intravenous infusion set (Courtesy Abbott Laboratories, North Chicago, Ill.)

closer to the proximal end of the limb tend to be larger than those situated more distally. However, even small veins can be used with careful attention to tourniquet application, dependent drainage, hand clenching by the patient and management of venous spasm.

ARMAMENTARIUM

If drugs are to be injected into the vein directly from a syringe, all that is needed is a 3- or 5-ml. syringe fitted with an 18- or 20-gauge needle (1½ inches long) plus alcohol sponges, adhesive bandages and a tourniquet. The needle point must be sharp and ground with a bevel of medium length. Long bevels are not easily threaded into veins. Commercially prepared tourniquets are available but a length of ¼-in. soft latex tubing will serve equally well.

The components of an infusion set include a bottle, or other reservoir, containing the solution to be administered, a drip chamber, a length of

tubing supplied with an adjustable flow rate control clamp, a latex injection site and a needle adapter to which is attached the same type of needle that would be placed on a syringe. The entire unit can be purchased in sterile disposable form.

The bottle, usually containing 5 per cent dextrose in water, is fitted with some means of hanging it inverted from a pole, an air inlet with filter fittings to receive the infusion tubing. The bottle is prepared by suspending it about 2 or 3 feet higher than the and opening the flow control to allow solution to run out a place all air in the tubing. With needle attached, this also ser test of needle patency.

Watching the rate at wh fall from the bottle into the ber permits observation of flow and will show if flow for any reason. If the becomes filled, this fu vented. To remedy this the flow clamp, take

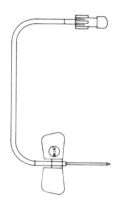

Fig. 50. Diagram representing the parts of a butterfly needle. (Courtesy Abbott Laboratories, North Chicago, Ill.)

turn it upright and then squeeze the drip chamber and force some solution back into the bottle.

The tubing serves as a conduit carrying solution from the reservoir to the needle. Here also are the means of controlling flow rate (adjustable clamp) and introducing drugs into the infusion (self-sealing latex injection site). The tubing is clear so that air bubbles or reflux of blood can be seen. The needle adapter is of standard size and design that will accept all needles. Should the tubing prove too short, sterile disposable extension tubes are available. Infusion sets are available with drip rates ranging from 10 drops per ml. up to about 60 drops per milliliter. For most cases a rate of about 20 drops per milliliter is best. Consult the package label for this information.

One variation in armamentarium that is preferred by some operators is the use of a butterfly needle. Instead of the standard hub, this type of needle is fitted with two flexible plastic wings, a short length of tubing (about 6 inches) and a female needle adapter. The wings are held folded together during venipuncture, allowing for more accurate manipulation and angulation of the needle more parallel to the skin. When the wings are laid flat after insertion they provide more secure anchoring surfaces for fixation to the skin and lessen chances of needle movement within the vein. The flexible tubing allows for connection to various syringes or infusion sets without disturbing the needle. After venipuncture and before removing the tourniquet, remove the cap from the end of the tubing (reflux of blood will clear the air from the tubing) before connecting it to the solution source.

The rate of flow of the infusion can be varied by adjustment of the clamp which, on different sets, may be of the pinch or screw variety. If the rate remains too slow, raise the bottle, warm the solution, check the needle position or start another infusion with a larger needle.

Properly assembled and started, few occurrences inhibit the flow of the infusion. If difficulty is encountered, check for a kink in the tubing, a clogged air inlet in the bottle or a displaced or obstructed needle.

The temperature of the solution is not critical, as a rather wide range will be tolerated by the patient. Dextrose in water, most commonly used, is stable at room temperature and need not be refrigerated. The small volume used will be quickly diluted and brought to the temperature of the circulating blood. Always read the container label before use and examine the solution to be sure that it is clear. The bottle and other parts of the infusion set should not be damaged in any way.

MANAGEMENT

By introducing drugs directly into the circulating blood we eliminate the need for absorption and greatly increase the rapidity of onset. Some sedative effect can be seen after a latent

period of only 20 to 25 sec. (the arm-brain circulation time). The level of depression can be precisely controlled since the dosage can be varied according to effect and empirical predetermination is not necessary. The desired degree of sedation can be maintained for extended periods by slow injection of small increments as they become necessary.

However, as in many situations, the same properties of the technique that may benefit the patient and operator carry with them the potential for dan-

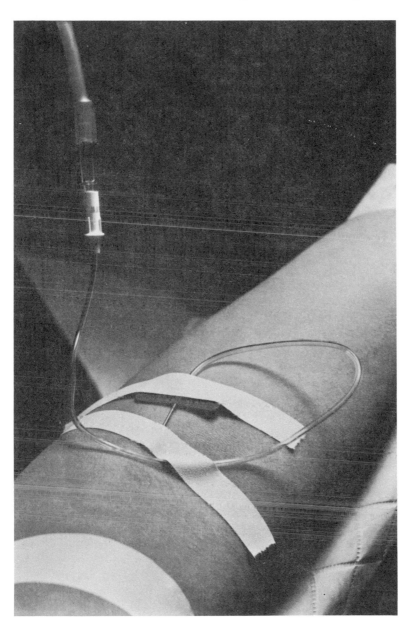

Fig. 51. The wings of a butterfly needle, when laid flat, provide a more secure anchoring surface for fixing the needle to the skin.

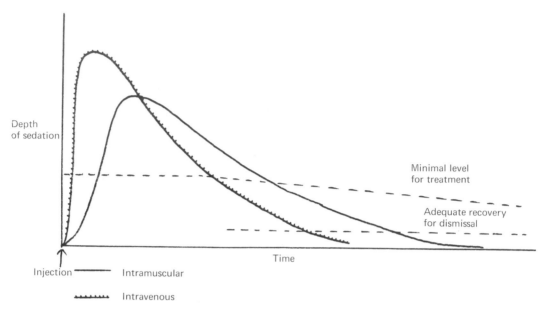

COMPARISON OF SEDATIVE EFFECT
FOLLOWING SINGLE INTRAMUSCULAR
AND INTRAVENOUS INJECTIONS

FIG. 52. After intravenous injection, the latent period before reaching effective sedative levels is shorter, the effect more pronounced and the recovery more rapid than after intramuscular injection of a similar dose.

ger. Rapid onset and induction may inadvertently predispose to rapid overdosage and unnecessarily and dangerously deep depression. No incremental doses should be injected until the effects of previous amounts have been determined. Contact with the patient must always be maintained by carefully and continuously monitoring vital signs.

The almost-supine contour chair position is probably the best for sedation cases. The head-low posture protects against cerebral hypotension. The slight upward angulation of the trunk aids vital capacity by eliminating pressure by the viscera against the underside of the diaphragm. Absence of a footrest prevents a patient who is entering excitement or dreaming from bracing his feet and creating force with his body. The widespread support for

the trunk and legs adds to a general feeling of comfort that enhances the effects of sedation. The doughnut type headrest allows for movement of the head and this facilitates operative access as well as airway maintenance. Finally, of course, this position has proven to be probably the most efficient one in which to perform dental procedures.

Intravenous drugs can be given either by the drip or surge methods. In the drip method the agent is added to the solution in the intravenous infusion bottle and the drip rate is adjusted so as to enter the venous circulation constantly but slowly. Control is attained by using extremely dilute solutions of drugs, and by careful attention to the effect on the patient. Periodic adjustments are made in the drip rate to maintain the patient at the

SEDATIVE EFFECT FOLLOWING A LARGE INITIAL DOSE
AUGMENTED WITH SMALLER SUBSEQUENT DOSES (INTRAVENOUSLY)

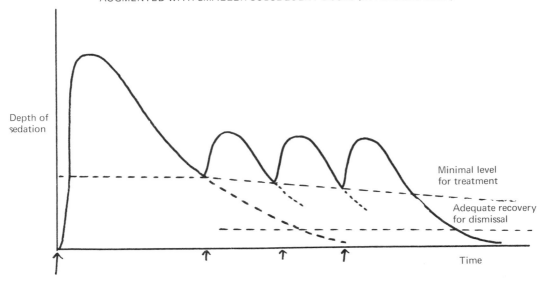

FIG. 53. As the sedative effect of the initial dose wanes, small additional intravenous surge doses will return the sedation to effective levels for periods of time shorter than after the original dose. Since the effects of previous doses are waning, the recovery curve will be steeper than that seen after the original larger dose. (Eventually, however, results from individual doses may show a cumulative effect as body reservoirs become saturated.)

desired level. With careful attention, this method can result in maintenance of the most precise and consistent levels of sedation even though measurement of the amount of drug injected is subject to some inaccuracy. The inflow of drug is balanced against lightening from drug detoxification or redistribution. If the operator's attention is divided, however, between anesthesia and operative procedures, there is the possibility of loss of constancy in sedative level. Depending upon the drip rate, the patient may inadvertently drift deeper or lighter.

In surge administration the drug enters the vein from a syringe only when it is consciously injected by the operator. Even though more concentrated solutions are used, control is attained through more accurate measurement of incremental doses and by injection of only small amounts at any given

time. Inattention may result in lack of administration of a dose necessary to maintain the proper level and the patient will drift lighter (but never deeper). Since the technique described here is one in which the dual functions of operator and anesthesiologist are performed by one person, surge administration is recommended because of this inherent safety factor.

One disadvantage of surge administration is the potential for blood clotting within the needle lumen between spaced injections. The clot could probably be forced out of the needle by pressure on the plunger but the ensuing embolus is as dangerous as one arising from any other cause. This danger is avoided by starting an infusion of dextrose and water and maintaining a constant slow drip throughout the case so that no clotting will occur in the needle. The minimal rate for this protection is about 1 drop every 5 seconds. Incremental surge injections are made from a syringe with its needle inserted through the gum rubber injection site in the infusion set. A small diameter needle (25 gauge) is preferable to the larger needle (18 to 20 gauge) needed for venipuncture since it will enter the tubing with less disturbance to the infusion set. Injection rate is adequate (even with the smaller needle) since the drug will be propelled forward by the plunger pressure which is greater than that derived by gravity in the infusion (requiring a larger needle). Aseptic technique must be followed during injection into the tubing.

For most purposes, sedation should be carried to the onset of cortical effect (drowsiness, dizziness, blurring of vision and thickened speech) and then one further small increment given. Further injections should be made as necessary to maintain this level.

Absence of dental pain must be ensured through use of local anesthesia. Painful stimuli will lessen the sedative effect. Once pain has been experienced it will take more drug to reestablish the sedative level than it would to produce the same result prior to the stimulation. Since local anesthetic injection can itself be painful, sedative effect must be well established before the intraoral injections. The size and frequency of incremental doses can be gauged from the response of the patient to the previous doses. As the case progresses the need for further increments decreases while previous amounts are losing their effect, and this fortuitous circumstance aids in avoiding overdosage and in shortening the recovery time before dismissal. As the body's reservoirs become saturated, less of each increment will be withdrawn from the circulating blood and more care is needed to avoid overdosage and excessive depression.

For these reasons intravenous dosage cannot be standardized. Each case exhibits its own characteristics and these will vary from time to time in a given management. There are certain yardsticks that will aid in gauging dosage, but these are not absolute and must be considered in light of the effect produced. Further, because of the instantaneous absorption, a definite time-dose relationship exists. The same dose if given more rapidly will saturate the tissues faster, producing a more profound effect and, possibly, will require a smaller total dose over the duration of the management. We are straddling a fine line though, because too much too soon can produce acute overdosage and may dangerously affect vital functions. There are no substitutes for careful technique and experience.

AGENTS

Dosage and Reactions

The controllability of intravenous sedation makes possible variant effects from the same drugs. Depth of sedation will vary with dosage and manner of injection. However, for practical purposes, some drugs are inherently less sedating, and production of deeper levels would require so much drug as to invite excessive side effects. On the other hand, for more moderate levels these drugs act well, since they do not impair vital functions if used in this manner. Some agents are preferable for moderate sedation and some for deeper effects.

MODERATE EFFECT
  Diazepam (Valium)
  Promethazine (Phenergan)

MORE PROFOUND EFFECT
  Secobarbital (Seconal)
  Pentobarbital (Nembutal)

  { Alphaprodine (Nisentil)
  { Levallorphan (Lorfan)

As a general rule, intravenous injections should be made slowly. This can be facilitated by diluting the solution or by injecting fractions of the dose separated by short intervals. Promethazine, for example, if used alone will probably require about 100 mg. to produce a pleasant, relaxed effect for most persons. Two ml. of a 50 mg. per ml. solution should be drawn into a syringe which is inserted, through the gum rubber injection site, into the tubing of the dextrose and water infusion. The promethazine should be injected in four portions of 25 mg. each, separated by at least 30 to 60 sec. Slowness of injection may be facilitated if several milliliters of sterile water for injection or 5 percent dextrose in water are drawn into the syringe to dilute the drug. Use of diluted solution in a larger syringe makes measurement easier.

The desired effect may be attained before the full 100 mg. has been given and, in that event, further administration is contraindicated. On the other hand, if by a few minutes after the last increment, sufficient sedation is still lacking, further small doses can be added with care and observance of proper precautions.

Diazepam (Valium) must be injected into the venous circulation extremely slowly. The usual dose of 10 mg. suffices for most adults. The ampule is opened and the 2 ml. of diazepam (5 mg. per ml.) is drawn into a 10 ml. syringe preparatory to dilution of the drug. Diazepam is incompatible with our common diluents (water, saline, dextrose in water), forming a dense cloudiness or precipitate in their presence. Only blood can be used to dilute the diazepam. The drug should be injected directly into the vein and not into an infusion.

After venipuncture and before removal of the tourniquet (blood is always removed while the tourniquet is still in place; solutions are never injected until after removal of the tourniquet), pull back on the plunger and aspirate approximately 8 ml. of blood into the syringe. Remove the tourniquet and slowly inject the diluted diazepam. (Clotting in the needle will not present a problem in the minute or two necessary for the injection.) Then, while firmly holding the needle hub, detach the syringe, attach the needle connector of the infusion set and start the dextrose infusion. The needle must be firmly fixed during these manipulations since sideways pressure or movement may force it through the walls of the vein. Butterfly needles, because of the short length of flexible tubing between the needle and female adapter, are best used in this technique. Movement at the needle adapter will not torque or twist the needle in the vein.

Because of reports of endarteritis, thrombosis and digital gangrene, the manufacturer has withdrawn its recommendation that hydroxyzine (Atarax, Vistaril) be administered intravenously. The company feels that these untoward occurrences were due to inadvertent intra-arterial injection, but this is only conjecture on its part. In the face of such a warning, the drug must *never* be used intravenously. Failure to heed the warning may well constitute malpractice. There has been no warning against intramuscular injection and, for that purpose, hydroxyzine remains an excellent agent.

For more profound sedation, the barbiturates secobarbital (Seconal) and pentobarbital (Nembutal) work well. The usual dose of either will be in the vicinity of 100 mg., which should be given in 25 mg. portions. The dose can be lessened or increased by 25 to 50 mg. as needed. Do not forget, though, that the barbiturates are among the most potent respiratory depressants. In subhypnotic doses profound respiratory depression is rarely seen but vigilance can never be relaxed. Mild depression is sometimes seen and the potential for more is always present. While the onset and duration of pentobarbital are longer than those of secobarbital, this distinction is much less evident with intravenous administration than with other routes. If the management is to be one hour or less, secobarbital is preferable. If more sedation is required after the case has progressed for some time, secobarbital should be used regardless of which of the two was given originally.

Narcotics may be used for sedation also. Alphaprodine (Nisentil) is effective and, because of its relatively short duration, is well suited for ambulatory dental management. An attempt to minimize its respiratory depressant effects is made by combination of the drug with the narcotic antagonist, levallorphan (Lorfan). Theoretically, the antagonist prevents the respiratory depression without altering the sedative capabilities of the narcotic. Curiously, the antagonist depresses respiration if it is administered to an unnarcotized patient or if its effect persists after recovery from the narcotic. The alphaprodine and levallorphan constitute an effective combination because their durations are (1 to 1½ hours intravenously) similar.

The proportion of one drug to the other is important and a special procedure should be followed in their measurement. Alphaprodine can be purchased in a multiple-dose vial in a strength of 60 mg./ml. Levallorphan is available in a 1 ml. ampule containing 1 mg. of drug. The mixture is made in a 30 ml. reusable vial of sterile saline for injection. Withdraw (and discard) 2 ml. of saline from the vial so that 28 ml. remains. Withdraw 0.9 ml. (54 mg.) of alphaprodine from its vial and inject this into the saline vial. Similarly, add the 1 ml. (1 mg.) of levallorphan to the saline. The restored 30 ml. (approximately) in the saline vial now contains 1.8 mg. of alphaprodine and 1/30 mg. of levallorphan per milliliter of solution.

Whenever the contents of a vial are modified you must relabel it to reflect the altered content. The label should include the amounts of all drugs contained in the bottle and the date of preparation. Always reread the label before use. The shelf life will be prolonged if the vial is refrigerated after each use.

For injection, withdraw 10 ml. of mixed solution into a syringe. The 18 mg. of alphaprodine and 1/3 mg. of levallorphan contained in the 10 ml. syringe constitutes the presumptive dose. This should be injected slowly into the infusion, observing the usual precautions for modification of dose according to observed effect. Increments of 2 to 3 ml. of the mixture can be used as necessary while the case progresses.

Atropine, in a dose of 1/150 gr. (0.4 mg.), may be given in addition to any of the sedative agents for its antisialogic properties. In general anesthetic management it is used also because its vagolytic properties are thought to lessen the incidence of laryngospasm (initiated by a vagal reflex), but this rationale lacks validity in sedative management. It has been our experience that, in a lengthy operative case, dryness (without atropine) is more apparent than salivary excess and that atropine is not needed. In any event, its use is contraindicated for patients with glaucoma, prostatic hypertrophy and asthma and, because of possible tachycardia, relatively contraindicated for hypertensives. Generally, it should not be given to patients older than forty years.

COMBINATIONS

Nitrous oxide analgesia complements intravenous sedation with all agents.

The analgesia may facilitate acceptance of the venipuncture. The movement of the breathing bag simplifies monitoring of respiratory function. The rapid deepening and lightening possible with nitrous oxide furnishes finer control over the total sedative effect. Intravenously administered sedation can be rapidly deepened but recovery is slower than the ultrarapid elimination of nitrous oxide. Use of nitrous oxide permits use of smaller amounts of the intravenous drugs, thereby accelerating recovery. However, it must be remembered that the intravenous and inhalation agents are adjuncts to local anesthesia and not substitutes for it. Adequate local anesthesia is mandatory for all sedative techniques. We can combine the various modes of medication to gain maximal advantage from each and to minimize their respective disadvantages.

The sedative drugs cited represent effective, safe agents for dental practice. They can be given in combination or other drugs can be used in their place. An experienced operator should be able to evaluate other methods and to manage safely their use on the basis of patient reaction, handling any unanticipated sequelae as they arise. Most experienced operators have their own preferences in sedative drugs

and almost any regimen can be safe and effective if used properly. The drugs presented here were chosen for introductory use. Promethazine will potentiate the sedative properties of the barbiturates but each must be injected from a separate syringe. Diazepam synergizes the alphaprodine/-levallorphan combination, but the differing methods of introduction for each must be adhered to. When drugs are used in combination, we can expect to reduce the dose of each. As the operator matures in sedative experience he can certainly graduate to use of other drug combinations.

In preparation for sedative practice, review venous anatomy and pharmacology. Plan the treatment procedure, considering the steps necessary in their normal sequence. Arrange the layout of equipment and supplies for convenient access and conduct a few dry runs to familiarize yourself with the sequence and to train your staff. Above all, select your initial patients carefully on the basis of accessibility of veins, physical constitution and only moderate need for sedation. Be prepared for occasional failures and do not allow pride to cloud your judgment and do not persist in unsuccessful attempts if difficulty arises.

15 | Treatment of Complications

In the practice of dentistry, as in all of life, conditions may occasionally arise which, if not eliminated or corrected, can promote discomfort or generate deleterious results that may compromise the future health and viability of various tissues or of the organism itself. With the oral or parenteral administration of centrally depressant drugs (sedative agents), further possibilities for difficulty are introduced and the potential danger is increased. Use of these modalities requires ability to recognize the occurrence and to treat effectively the manifestations of complications as they arise before they develop to a point of crisis.

Fortunately, with astute preoperative evaluation, careful utilization of methods and agents according to accepted principles and continuously meticulous observation of the patient's status, few true emergencies are experienced. Recognition of signs presaging difficulties makes it possible to decrease chances of their occurrence and lessen their severity.

Unfortunately, since emergency situations are rare, the opportunity to learn their management through practice and repetition is limited. Skill in full crown preparation can be attained and refined by preparing many teeth over an extended period of time, but a cardiac arrest in a dental office will, most likely, be the first any member of the operating team has ever seen. The capability for successful treatment of complications must come from study of the characteristics of agents and methods and practice in the sequence of steps to be undertaken. Practice drills for simulated emergencies can extend the training to the office staff. Rarely, when faced with an urgent situation, will we be afforded the luxury of time to consult a reference source or relay instructions to ancillary personnel. The dentist and the members of his staff must each be conversant with emergency procedures.

GENERAL PRINCIPLES

The basic principles to be followed relate to prevention and use of symptomatic supportive therapy rather than to reliance on specific antidotal drugs. Before using any sedative agent, familiarize yourself with the untoward sequelae that may result so you can adopt a procedure that skirts these possibilities. Adequate ventilatory exchange is mandatory and, when lacking, predisposes to various other problems. Cultivate the ability to maintain airway and ventilatory exchange in all situations.

The use of antidotal or corrective drugs should be relegated to a secondary role in treatment of complications. If respiration is depressed, assisted ventilation is therapeutic regardless of the cause, but if drugs are used there must first be a rather specific diagnosis of the cause. The dosage, too, must be carefully determined. Often, overdosage of corrective drugs leads to additional, and possibly more severe, complications. The attention required for diagnosis and preparation and administration of drugs can be distract-

148

ing, hence, counterproductive in an urgent situation.

RESPIRATORY COMPLICATIONS

Any interference with normal ventilatory function represents potential danger, since the body cannot store oxygen and must constantly have access to a fresh supply. There are likewise no mechanisms for carbon dioxide breakdown and since accumulation leads to untoward sequelae, the capability for adequate respiratory elimination must be present at all times.

Total failure of ventilatory capability whether due to severe anesthetic depression, airway obstruction by foreign matter or vomitus in the pharynx or aspirated into the tracheobronchial tree, laryngeal or bronchial spasm, soft tissue occlusion of the airway, or from any other cause represents a grave emergency as permanent brain damage occurs after as little as 3 to 5 minutes of absolute lack of cerebral oxygen supply. Inadequate cerebral oxygenation may result from such causes as lack of carbon dioxide to stimulate the respiratory center, hypoxia that depresses that center, drug depression, excitation of various reflex mechanisms that only partially adduct the vocal cords or constrict the bronchioles. Subtotal mechanical obstruction, partial loss of airway patency from tongue or head position presents a less critical emergency but, nevertheless, it requires corrective and supportive measures to avoid inadequate cerebral oxygen levels that can cause gradual damage and depress vital centers to the point where more urgent conditions supervene.

Basically, the treatment of respiratory embarrassment involves steps to augment ventilation and to eliminate the causes of inadequacy. Any drugs or agents previously given should immediately be suspect and further administration should cease. Airway pa-

tency should be checked and improved if necessary. This can be done by extending the head to straighten the airway, protruding the mandible by anteriorly directed pressure behind the gonial angles in order to pull the tongue forward out of the pharynx, and the head turned to the side so that foreign matter or vomitus collects in the cheek rather than in the pharynx. Vomitus, debris, mucus, blood or other small bits of material in the mouth and pharynx should be suctioned out with care to avoid stimulating the laryngeal reflexes which might cause laryngospasm and would greatly intensify the urgency of the situation. Similarly, a nasal or oral airway cannot usually be inserted in the patient who is sedated (however heavily) but who is not asleep, since the pharyngeal and laryngeal reflexes are not obtunded and the danger exists of creating an even greater emergency. Oxygen should be administered under positive pressure either in pure form from an anesthesia machine through a face mask or, lacking such equipment, by means of mouth-to-mouth or mouth-to-nose artificial respiration. The chest should expand during artificial respiration and if it does not, the steps for improving the airway should be repeated. If the patient is making some spontaneous inspiratory effort, the artificial augmentation should be in synchrony with these attempts and should never counter them. Artificial assistance of ventilation should be continued until the need for it no longer exists.

Support of Respiration
1. Cease administration of agents
2. Improve airway
   Remove obstructing matter
   Relieve anatomic obstruction
3. Administer oxygen

These procedures are of foremost importance and of greatest value. Use of drugs to stimulate respiration are of less value and should be subordinated to a secondary role or avoided as being of questionable benefit in most cases. Certain specific conditions merit further elucidation.

Dyspnea

Dyspnea is a state of difficult or labored breathing in an awake patient. The patient is aware of the respiratory distress and will often inform the operator of its occurrence.

The etiology of dyspnea often involves cerebral impulses arising as a result of anxiety and apprehension, reflex mechanisms or mechanical interference with respiration as from pressure upon the chest wall or abdominal viscera pressing upward against the diaphragm and impeding its downward inspiratory movement.

Treatment entails removal of the causes by cessation of pressure on the chest, positioning the trunk at a slight upward angle so the abdominal viscera fall away from the diaphragm, verbal reassurance, moderate sedation to allay apprehension and promote relaxation, and administration of an oxygen-enriched gas mixture (possible oxygen-rich air) to make embarrassed ventilation more efficacious. Dyspnea, if untreated, tends to become progressively worse as a vicious cycle is established; apprehension begets dyspnea which frightens the patient, and makes for further dyspnea.

Hypoxia

Hypoxia is the state in which the tissues fail to receive or utilize physiologically adequate amounts of oxygen. (Anoxia denotes total oxygen lack.) There are several basic etiologic mechanisms causing hypoxia and each has been given its own name.

Hypoxic hypoxia involves suboxygenation of arterial blood due to inspiration of inadequate amounts of oxygen as from too low a percentage of oxygen in the inspired mixture, depressed respiration or a partially obstructed airway. *Anemic hypoxia* results from a diminished oxygen-carrying capacity of the blood due possibly to a shortage of hemoglobin; this can occur during anemia or after severe hemorrhage. *Stagnant hypoxia* follows from inability of the circulatory system to distribute the oxygen carried within it as from shock, impaired venous return, or any circulatory failure of cardiac origin. *Histotoxic hypoxia* results from tissue damage that renders the cells incapable of utilizing oxygen made available to them. *Diffusion hypoxia* is an anesthesiologist's concept; this can be the situation after cessation of nitrous oxide administration wherein the gas diffuses out of the blood so rapidly as to create such a high tension in the lungs as to prevent entrance of oxygen during inspiration. *Metabolic hypoxia* is a relative condition in which the metabolism is so increased as to outstrip the body's capacity to deliver oxygen even in the absence of depression. Causes may include such conditions as unreasonable fear, elevated body temperature or induction excitement.

Coping with hypoxia deals with both prevention and remediation. If anemia is suspected and confirmed by laboratory data, elective sedation (used for the majority of dental procedures) should be deferred and the patient treated by other means. The case should be cancelled if there is cardiac decompensation or febrile disease. Patency of the airway should be checked and improved to eliminate obstruction. If respiration is pharmacologically depressed, no further agents should be administered. Oxygen flow rates should be increased, cylinders checked for depletion and ventilation augmented where indicated. At the close of the management, large amounts of oxygen should be used to wash out nitrous oxide from the anesthetic system. Additional sedation can be given to alleviate apprehension if excessive amounts which cause depression have not already been administered.

Constant vigilance is necessary to guard against establishment of an hypoxic state. The first signs may be increased pulse and respiratory rates. Later, the pulse may be slow and strong with elevated systolic pressure and, still later, as cardiac muscle is depressed, the pulse tends to be slow and weak with the possibilty of arrhythmia. As hypoxia progresses there may be muscular rigidity and tremors with increased motor activity, much like that seen in the excitement stage. Depression resulting from oxygen lack may lessen respiratory activity as the hypoxia becomes more severe and, in the ultimate situation, circulatory collapse and cardiac arrest may occur.

Cyanosis often appears as a warning sign and is best visualized in the lips, face and nail beds. It must be remembered, though, that cyanosis is a symptom not of oxygen lack but of the presence of excessive amounts of reduced hemoglobin so that in relatively anemic persons it may not be seen. In extremely florid persons the amount of reduced hemoglobin may be too small percentage-wise to produce a visible effect and in dark-skinned patients relatively advanced cyanosis may be masked by the skin color.

Obstructed Respiration

Respiratory obstruction can be partial or complete, centered in the upper or lower respiratory tract areas, extrinsically produced as from foreign body impaction or be of intrinsic physiological origin as is seen with laryngospasm or bronchiolar constriction. The degree of urgency is related to the degree of obstruction. Total obstruction must be treated before 3 or 4 minutes have elapsed.

The first evidence of obstruction is interference with the normal sequential pattern of inspiration and expiration. With lesser obstruction, respiratory smoothness disappears and the patient is apt to gasp, cough, gag or wheeze. Inspiratory effort can be prolonged with attendant slowing of the respiratory rate. In severe obstruction, gases cannot enter normally, the equalization of intrathoracic negative pressure is blocked and the chest does not expand. With the sternum retracting and the diaphragm pulled upward by the intrathoracic negative pressure, the abdomen is sucked in and a characteristic rocking motion is seen.

If the situation is untreated, hypoxia progresses to anoxia and the symptoms become those of asphyxiation. Central nervous system centers are depressed and vital functions deteriorate.

Upper tract obstruction. Obstruction of the upper tract (nasal passages, oral cavity, nasal and oral pharynx) can result from a poorly placed anesthetic mask, poor head position such as a sharp sideways rotation or extreme ventral flexion of the neck (mandible depressed to the point where it nears or touches the anterior chest wall), relaxation of the pharyngeal walls so that they fall in leaving a smaller space within, posterior relaxation of the tongue allowing it to fall back into the pharynx, or materials in the mouth and pharynx whether they be a poorly placed pharyngeal partition, debris of dental treatment, blood or vomitus.

Management of respiratory obstruction is related to the prevention of precipitating factors as well as their remediation. Careful technique prevents occurrence of most obstruction. The head should be firmly supported in a

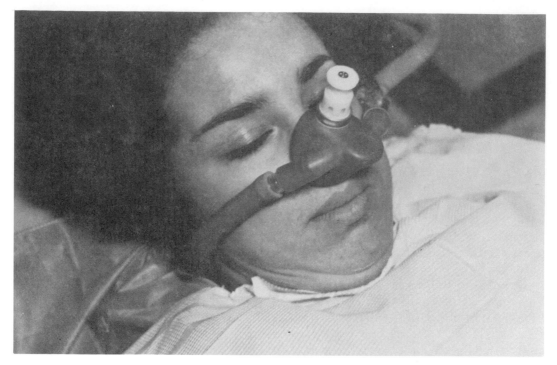

FIG. 54. Incorrect position of the head (chin against the chest) can compromise the patency of the airway and lead to respiratory embarrassment.

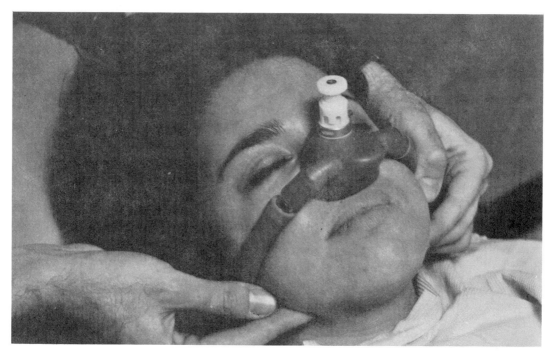

FIG. 55. The airway can often be improved if the head is extended and the mandible protruded by anteriorly directed pressure behind the gonial angles.

nearly postural relationship to the trunk with perhaps slight dorsal flexion of the neck and with no lateral rotation. Soft tissue relaxation is not profound enough to compromise the airway in patients only lightly sedated but in deeper levels this can pose a problem. Anteriorly directed pressure maintains the mandible in a protruded position and this helps to draw the tongue out of the pharynx.

Aspiration of matter through the larynx and into the lower respiratory tract is unlikely to occur in patients maintained in an awake sedated state. However, debris falling back into the pharynx can cause coughing and gagging, seriously hampering the operator. A pharyngeal screen (a 3 x 3-inch gauze square with a string attached) will prevent particles or liquids from falling back but can, of itself, create problems if improperly inserted. The partition should be draped over the forefinger and inserted in an arc following the palate and directed over the dorsum of the tongue. Improperly placed, the partition can push the tongue back and, if inserted too far, can cause gagging on its own.

If the patient has eaten nothing, vomiting does not pose a great problem for aspiration, since it consists only of gastric juice with no solid particles and is easily suctioned.

The anesthetic equipment should be checked before beginning the management and rechecked periodically during the case to be certain that gases are flowing unimpeded. The nasal mask should be of sufficient size so as not to compress the nares and should be centrally placed over the nose with sufficient tightness to maintain its position but without excessive tension that could flatten it and cause obstruction.

Laryngospasm. Closure of the vocal cords can be triggered as a protective reflex mechanism intended to prevent the passage of foreign matter through the larynx and into the trachea and bronchi. During sedation, the cough reflex can be dulled and foreign matter may be tolerated long enough for irritation of the larynx to activate the reflex through stimulation of the vagal innervation of the vocal cords. Care is particularly essential during use of sub-hypnotic doses of barbiturates which may sensitize the reflex.

Foreign particles or liquid should be carefully suctioned from the pharynx so that they will not be exciting factors and to prevent stimulation of the cords by the suction tip. Premedication with atropine (1/150 grain for an adult) is frequently used for its vagolytic action and for the reduction of possible salivary accumulation, but the effectiveness of this method is open to debate as only the serous portion of salivary production is deterred and the resultant viscid saliva may be more difficult to evacuate and more likely to adhere to and stimulate the vocal cords. A dose of 1/150 grain of atropine is felt by some to be too small for truly effective depression of the vagal tone but larger doses may have untoward sequelae such as pronounced tachycardia and heat retention.

Sedation should be postponed for any patient exhibiting an inflammatory condition of the tissues of the airway. In all persons manipulation of the tissues and of the mandible and head should be as gentle as possible.

Partial adduction of the vocal cords may be diagnosed by the presence of inspiratory stridor (a harsh, vibratory sound) or by crowing. With complete closure of the cords, the symptoms are those of total obstruction and anoxia. Treatment of partial spasm includes relief of anatomic obstruction of the airway, evacuation of the pharynx and administration of oxygen under positive pressure. During total spastic closure of the cords, oxygenation will be impossible. Manual compression of the thorax repeated several times may force out obstructing matter from the cords but if this is unsuccessful surgical establishment of an airway by cricothyrostomy should be considered. Some laryngospasms will be broken spontaneously as anoxia develops but this is not to be relied upon.

Use of muscle relaxant drugs, by paralyzing the musculature of the vocal cords, will cause them to relax and allow oxygen to pass, but this method should be reserved for clinicians prepared to intubate the trachea and to treat the respiratory arrest resulting from total flaccid paralysis of all body skeletal muscles. In untrained hands, this condition can be a more grave threat to life than the original laryngospasm. Also, relaxation of the cords (with vigorous oxygenation) may allow aspiration of the foreign body originally responsible for the spasm.

Bronchial spasm. Like laryngospasm, contraction of the bronchial or bronchiolar musculature can cause embarrassment of ventilatory function with the degree of urgency related to the degree of muscular spasm. Possible causes likewise include vagal and mechanical stimulation. Unlike laryngospasm, the obstruction occurs not at one point but along the length of the tubes and the muscle fibers involved are smooth rather than striated. (Muscle relaxant drugs are totally without effect and useless in treatment.) Persons suffering from chronic pulmonary disease, asthma or hereditary allergies are more likely to experience bronchial spasm so that in such patients this type of management might best be avoided.

Because the bronchial lumens are narrowed, expulsion of air from the lungs is impeded and the expiratory portion of the respiratory cycle is prolonged. Patients breathe with a characteristic asthmatic wheezing sound, the chest may be distended and, in severe cases, cyanosis may be evident.

A mild attack may be treated with just airway management and oxygen administration. In severe cases, bronchodilating drugs should be used. First, inject ¼ to ½ ml. of 1:1000 epinephrine subcutaneously. (Repeat in 20 minutes if necessary.) This can be followed with ¼ to ½ gram of aminophylline injected intravenously. (Inject slowly—it may cause marked hypotension.) The patient should be hydrated intravenously with 500 ml. of 5 percent dextrose in water and, if the attack remains intractible, medical consultation should be sought promptly. In some cases, sedation with 50 to 100 mg. of pentobarbital (Nembutal) intravenously (avoiding respiratory depression) will calm the patient and make him more comfortable, since the need for oxygen decreases with quiescence. A corticosteroid such as Solu-Cortef (100 mg. intravenously) is recommended by some but is of less immediate benefit.

Procedures for relieving obstruction. Relief of obstruction begins with its recognition and proceeds from quicker, simpler procedures to the more involved. The patient should always be watched for such signs as gasping, coughing, wheezing, choking, suprasternal retraction and cyanosis. Diagnosis is simplified if a foreign body has just been seen to disappear into the pharynx.

A diligent (but gentle) attempt should be made to remove foreign matter, the head should be lowered, the airway should be improved as much as possible by extending the head, protruding the mandible and, possibly, grasping the tongue and pulling it forward. (A pharyngeal airway should not be inserted in an awake patient, as it may aggravate gagging.) Management is usually simpler during sedation than with general anesthesia because the patient is making a voluntary respiratory effort and might cough up an offending particle. Oxygen should be administered under positive pressure synchronous with the patient's efforts.

If all attempts to ventilate a patient are unsuccessful, an emergency surgical airway can be created by opening through the cricothyroid membrane (cricothyrostomy) in the neck. This membrane connects the thyroid cartilage (Adam's apple) with the next inferior cartilage, the cricoid. There are no important structures or vessels superficial to this membrane so that surgical access is uncomplicated and bleeding is slight.

Palpation of the membrane below the prominence of the laryngeal cartilage is easier with the neck flexed and incision is more efficiently accomplished with the neck stretched. Palpate the position of the membrane and, keeping a finger over the spot, extend the neck. Make a ½-in. transverse incision across the midline of the neck while fixing the larynx with digital pressure. Patients will often cough as the trachea is entered and a rush of air may be heard. The opening should be kept patent by inserting a rubber tube that can be fixed to the skin to prevent dislodgement or entry into the trachea. A special curved metal tube (cannula) with a pointed stylet (trocar) and wings for skin fixation is available. This procedure is for acute emergency treatment and not suitable for prolonged use. Medical assistance should be sought for continued care.

In the acute emergency situation, time is more important than asepsis, hemostasis or regional anesthesia. Infection and cartilage damage may result but these sequelae are certainly more manageable than death!

CARDIOVASCULAR COMPLICATIONS

Heart Rate and Rhythm

In a normal healthy person the heart rate and rhythm remain relatively constant, but it must be remembered that patients are not machines and that some transient variations will occur that do not threaten the safety or well-being of the patient. As long as the variations remain within certain limits, we observe and note their occurrence but do not necessarily take remedial action.

Heart rate in a frightened, nervous person would be expected to be faster than for the same person in a calm state. Not until the adult rate exceeds 100 per minute should it be considered *tachycardia*. Other causes, in addition to apprehension, are induction excitement, overdose of sympathomimetic or parasympatholytic drugs, hypoxia or painful stimulation. Attention should be paid to adequate premedication or comedication, local anesthesia, ventilation and judicious use of atropine or other belladonna drugs. The surroundings should be carefully controlled to prevent untoward or excessive distractive stimulation. One advantage of sedative management is the absence of induction excitement since the patient remains in the analgesia stage and is never carried to that point of depth.

Bradycardia, or heart rate slower than 60 per minute, is occasionally associated with hypoxia or with vagal stimulation. Atropine is most commonly used to combat vagal effects but the dosage and efficacy are subject to debate. With the onset of sedative relaxation, some slowing of the heart is frequently seen but this usually represents a return to the normal nonanxious base line rather than bradycardia, and often is more desirable than not.

Arrhythmia, or a departure from the normal rhythm of the heartbeat, can impair cardiac function if it is severe enough. It is more commonly seen in persons with some form of preexisting heart disease but can become apparent in anyone as a result of hypoxia, carbon dioxide accumulation, vagal reflexes or effects of inhalation agents. In general, the more irregular the arrhythmia the more profound is its implication but, in basically healthy persons, even relatively marked transient arrhythmias can be reversed by elimination of the causes. As in so many other complications, the important points are recognition and early management. Failure to treat arrhythmia can impair cardiac filling and output, leading to hypotension and reduced coronary artery flow.

Since hypoxia and carbon dioxide retention are common predisposing factors, care should be directed toward maintenance of airway and proper ventilation. Nitrous oxide will not markedly affect the myocardium as can other inhalation anesthetics and, for this reason, this technique is limited to the use of this agent. Even nitrous oxide should be discontinued if the arrhythmia continues. Patients with serious cardiac disease should be sedated only with extreme care, by persons adequately trained, and then only in situations where back-up emergency facilities are available.

Blood Pressure

Hypertension, or elevated blood pressure, can be brought on by apprehension, painful stimuli or hypoxia (with carbon dioxide retention). Patients must be evaluated beforehand to determine their individual tolerance and then adequately treated to avoid painful stimulation, and to produce sedative relaxation. Sedation may be particularly indicated for patients who are normally relatively hypertensive to prevent sudden acute rises that may predispose to emergent complications. Inhalation of amyl nitrate, a sympathetic blocking agent, is helpful in lowering blood pressure.

Hypotension, subnormal blood pressure, is often drug-related with the causative factors being possibly overdose of anesthetic agents or previous pharmacological management. Patients with a history of hypotension, poorly compensated cardiac insufficiency, endocrine dysfunction or anemia are particularly susceptible. In any patient, hypoxia and carbon dioxide excess, after initially producing hypertension, gradually lead to hypotension. Profuse bleeding (probably not often seen in dental treatment) may also be a causative factor.

Effects of recent therapy with hypotensive drugs can be synergized by excessive anesthetic depression or even moderate amounts of the phenothiazine group of tranquilizers. Interaction between central nervous system depressants (particularly narcotics) and the mono-amine oxidase (MOA) inhibitors, a group of antidepressant drugs (whether patients are currently taking them or have previously), can lead to a serious drop in blood pressure. The effects of these drugs persist for a substantial period following discontinuation of therapy. Patients who have been on a regimen of corticosteroid therapy may manifest adrenal insufficiency and, if the steroids are withdrawn before treatment, hypotension may ensue.

Diagnosis can be presumed on the basis of a pallid, ashen appearance and confirmed, of course, by taking the blood pressure. All anesthesia should be stopped, the patient placed flat and oxygen administered. Any hypotensive episode, whatever the cause, carries the potential for developing into a serious emergency, so treatment must begin promptly. Lifting the legs causes the blood contained within them (possibly

> MONO-AMINE OXIDASE INHIBITORS
> Nardil (phenelzine sulfate)
> Niamid (nialamide)
> Parnate (tranylcypromine)
> Marplan (isocarboxazid)
> Eutonyl (pargyline HCl)
>
> Plus some stimulants:
>
> Cocaine
> Benzedrine (amphetamine)
> Dexedrine (dexamphetamine)
> Methedrine (methamphetamine)
> Preludin (phenmetrazine)
> Ephedrine

a pint in each leg) to drain back to the trunk and has a hypertensive effect similar to blood transfusion. If there is no blood pressure improvement a vasopressor should be given (with care to prevent elevation above normal). Wyamine (mephentermine), given in a dose of 15 to 30 mg. intramuscularly or intravenously, is an effective vasopressor that is among the least likely to produce rebound hypertension. Any vasopressor given to a patient on MOA inhibitors may produce an exaggerated response. If the hypotension still persists, suspect adrenal cortical insufficiency and give 100 mg. of Solu-Cortef (hydrocortisone) intravenously.

Syncope, Shock

Syncope represents a sudden loss of consciousness from cerebral ischemia due to pooling of blood in other areas, while shock involves a more generalized inadequacy of circulating blood volume presenting a more serious eventuality and demanding more urgent treatment.

Syncope (fainting) can occur to anyone at any time and is most commonly caused in dental offices by psychogenic factors such as fear and apprehension. By recognizing prodromal symptoms such as pallor, sweating, nausea, dizziness and malaise, treatment can be instituted before loss of consciousness occurs and the onset can be reversed and a total faint prevented. By establishing rapport with the patient, we can instill confidence and allay the apprehension that can lead to syncope. Sedation, perhaps just nitrous oxide analgesia, can reduce nervousness. Instruments should be kept out of sight, waiting should be minimal and the environment made as pleasant and nonthreatening as possible.

Should the symptoms appear, the patient should be laid flat (possibly with the legs elevated), oxygen given, a cold towel applied to the forehead and constricting clothing loosened. Reflex stimulation by inhalation of aromatic spirits of ammonia is beneficial. Should consciousness be lost, the airway must be protected. Recurrence is always a possibility so the patient should be observed, reassured and continue to lie supine for a few minutes. A continuing feeling of nausea, if present, is often lessened by inhalation of oxygen for a short while.

Shock represents a more generalized circulatory embarrassment, perhaps resulting from any of several causes such as hemorrhagic decrease in volume of circulating blood, diminished cardiac output and hypotension as from cardiac failure or neurogenic (often psychogenic) vasodilation with diminished vasoconstrictor tone allowing blood to pool and be withdrawn from the effective circulation. The blood pressure drops, tissues can become ischemic, coronary flow suffers and a progressively worsening cycle can become established.

The signs of shock include pale, cold, moist skin, greyish, ashen cyanosis, thready, weak pulse, markedly decreased blood pressure and loss of consciousness. The major goal of emergency treatment is to counter or remove the causative factors and administer supportive therapy. All anesthesia should cease and the patient should be laid supine with the legs elevated. The airway should be protected and oxygen administered. The patient should be kept warm and hydrated with intravenous fluids (500 to 1000 ml. of 5 percent dextrose in water). A vasopressor such as Wyamine (mephentermine) can be given intravenously or intramuscularly in a dose of 15 to 30 mg. Local anesthetics can be given to relieve pain, if present, but narcotics should be avoided. Medical consultation should be promptly sought and hospitalization considered.

Cardiac Arrest

Cessation of cardiac function (asystole) accompanied, as it is, by pulmonary failure requires immediate action, since all cerebral oxygen will be depleted in as short a period as 10 seconds. After that time, destruction of brain tissue begins until, after about 4 minutes, vital centers are irreversibly destroyed and no recovery is possible. Recovery of heart function after shorter periods of cerebral ischemia can result in permanent mental and physiological impairment.

Possible causes are hypoxia from impaired ventilation or circulation, excessive chemical depression of the myocardium as from anesthetic agents or carbon dioxide, adverse reaction to drugs or rampant hypotension as from diminished venous return or loss of blood.

The onset is usually sudden but may be preceded by hypotension. Pulse and heart sounds are absent, respiration ceases, cyanosis persists even with artificial respiration, the skin acquires a yellowish waxlike appearance, bleeding usually stops (but may persist for a short while as veins drain) and the pupils are widely dilated and unresponsive to light.

Major treatment is to maintain artificial respiration and circulation in order to preserve the viability of the brain and vital organs. Secondarily, we attempt to restore spontaneous respiration and circulatory function. Cardiac muscle excitability increases in the first 3 to 4 minutes after arrest and then rapidly decreases to zero within 8 minutes. Chances of success are poor after 3 to 4 minutes without treatment, which would be of little value since, by then, irreversible brain damage would have occurred.

The patient should be ventilated with oxygen under positive pressure or mouth-to-mouth breathing and the oxygenated blood should be pumped through the circulatory system by rhythmically pressing on the lower third of the sternum. Flexibility of the costal cartilages allows compression of the anterior chest wall (the unconscious patient is relaxed) and the heart, sandwiched between the sternum and vertebral column, will be squeezed and its blood forced out. Enough oxygenated blood flow (40 to 60 percent of normal) may be obtained for maintaining viability of the heart and brain for as long as an hour if adequate cardiopulmonary support can be maintained for that period.

Cardiopulmonary resuscitation (external cardiac massage plus artificial respiration) should be begun as soon as arrest is suspected and even before confirmation. The procedure is a strenuous one and apt quickly to fatigue a single person so a team of two or even three persons is preferable.

The patient should be moved to a hard, unyielding surface such as the floor (a dental chair is seldom satisfactory), all appliances or foreign matter removed from the airway, the neck extended and the mandible protruded. Using mouth-to-mouth (or mouth-to-nose) breathing, breathe 3 or 4 times, watching to see that the patient's chest rises. Then, kneeling beside the patient, place the heel of one hand (fingers parallel to the ribs but not touching the chest) over the lower third of the sternum just above the xiphoid process, place the other hand on top of the first and exert a firm, downward pressure, depressing the sternum 1½ to 2 inches. Pause and hold the pressure at the end of the downstroke for a brief instant (while the heart empties) and quickly raise the hands, allowing the heart to refill. For frail individuals or large children use one hand. For small children use only several fingers. After each four compressions, inflate the lungs once, maintaining a pattern of 50 to 60 strokes and 12 to 15 inflations per minute.

Mouth-to-mouth artificial respiration is accomplished by clearing the airway, pinching the nostrils closed, placing the mouth fully over the patient's mouth and blowing with sufficient force to see the chest rise. After each breath, remove the mouth, turn away and take a deep breath. Mouth-to-nose breathing is performed similarly except that the mouth is held closed. Oxygen administered by positive pressure through a full face mask is desirable or an Ambu-type resuscitator can be used, but mouth-to-mouth breathing serves adequately if resuscitative equipment is not available.

A teamwork approach is best with one person compressing the chest and a second breathing for the patient, but one person alone can do a satisfactory job for a short while. In any event, the chest compression and lung inflation should be alternated so as not to counteract each other. A third person

can be of use to call for help, keep track of the time, raise the patient's legs, start an intravenous infusion (a difficult procedure with veins collapsed in the absence of blood pressure), administer drugs and feel for a peripheral pulse.

Epinephrine can be given intracardially (3 to 5 ml. of a 1:10,000 solution), repeated at 5-minute intervals, through a 3½-inch 22-gauge needle inserted into either ventricle through the fourth intercostal space. Dextrose 5 percent in water intravenously should be given rapidly. Epinephrine (1 to 2 ml. of a 1:10,000 solution) or Neo-synephrine (0.4 mg.) can be given intravenously followed by 100 mg. of Solu-Cortef.

If the resuscitation is effective, a carotid pulse should be detectable, the color should improve and the pupils should begin to contract and react to light. The patient may gasp, begin to breathe spontaneously, move his limbs and regain consciousness.

It is possible that one or more ribs will be fractured or the liver lacerated, but the possibility of these sequelae should not deter the operators from their tasks. In any event, medical assistance should be promptly sought, the patient kept under close observation and transferred to a hospital at the first opportunity. Cardiopulmonary resuscitation can be continued as he is transported.

Allergy

Any drug can be potentially allergenic with the most common manifestation being skin reaction such as urticaria (hives) or rash. Respiratory embarrassment or cardiovascular failure are possible sequelae but are rare with prompt treatment. Most often the major complaints are fever, malaise and itching. Speed of onset and rapidity of progression are the keys to determining seriousness. If the onset is more gradual, the danger is less, but if the symptoms develop rapidly a more severe reaction should be anticipated.

For a mild reaction, developing after some time-lapse and progressing slowly, the treatment is essentially symptomatic and seldom requires more than Benadryl (diphenhydramine) administered orally in doses of 25 to 50 mg., three to four times daily for adults and 10 to 20 mg., three to four times daily for children (Benadryl elixir—10 mg. per 4 ml.). Immediate intramuscular injection of the Benadryl is indicated for more profound symptoms.

A severe reaction begins almost immediately and represents a true emergency. A tourniquet should be applied proximal to the injection site (if intramuscular), 1:1000 epinephrine injected (0.5 ml. subcutaneously into the other arm repeated as necessary and 0.5 ml. intramuscularly into the initial injection site distal to the tourniquet). This can be followed with 25 to 50 mg. of Benadryl intramuscularly or intravenously and 100 mg. of Solu-Cortef intravenously (in the arm without the tourniquet). The patient should be laid supine, the airway protected, oxygen administered and medical help requested.

Epinephrine is given in the other arm because it has a direct antagonizing effect on histamine and at the initial injection site distal to the tourniquet it slows absorption of any of the offending agent that may remain. Certainly, no more of the allergenic drug should be given to that patient. Definitive determination of allergy can be obtained by referring the patient to an allergist for confirmatory testing.

With severe allergic reactions there is the possibility of circulatory failure and this, should it occur, takes precedence over all other conditions. The patient should be supine with the legs elevated and an intravenous infusion begun if it has not already been started. Aromatic spirits of ammonia should be used in an attempt to stimulate the patient and oxygen be given. If the blood pressure falls precipitously, Wyamine (mephentermine) should be given intramuscularly or, preferably, intravenously in a dose of 15 to 30 mg. in addition to the previously mentioned Benadryl and epinephrine. If no pulse is discernible, cardiopulmonary resuscitation must be begun immediately.

The barbiturates, so often used for sedation, seldom cause allergy and the shorter acting the drug the less likely it is to occur. Allergy to Nembutal and Seconal is, fortunately, rare. Reactions, when they do occur, are usually limited to a mild, transitory rash which disappears rapidly even if untreated. A more persistent rash can be treated with Benadryl.

DELAYED RECOVERY

The most common cause of delayed recovery is overdosage (a relative concept), caused perhaps by inaccurate assessment of the patient's needs, unanticipated susceptibility to the drugs, mistaken identity or strength of injected solutions, or cumulative effect of repeated injections. With proper care in handling solutions and correct technique (injection of small doses and assessment of the result before further administration), this should not occur.

Every label on every bottle or vial should be read before use and each syringe labelled as to its contents. Patients should be sedated with the minimal amount consistent with production of adequate quiescence needed for the operative procedure. This is accomplished by giving small increments and ascertaining the effect produced before continuing. Once the desired level is attained, no more agent should be given until such time as the patient becomes lighter. Since barbiturates and narcotics depress respiratory activity, observation of this function serves as a useful parameter in determining depth.

Treatment consists mainly of supportive measures and these include maintenance of blood pressure and adequate ventilation. Use of analeptic drugs is not the method of choice and should be considered only when other methods fail since there is the chance of producing further rebound effect later (e.g., vomiting, cardiac arrhythmias or convulsions). The effectiveness of these drugs is related to the degree of drug depression and may not be adequate to counter deep depression. Analeptics may further depress a respiratory center already depressed by hypoxia and should be used only in situations of depression caused by drug action.

Respiratory depression from overdose of narcotics can be countered with Nalline (nalorphine) given intravenously or intramuscularly in a dose of 5 to 10 mg. and repeated twice, if necessary, after 15-minute intervals. Nalline should be used only to counter narcotics, since it may actually depress respiration and circulation when given to an unnarcotized patient. Ritalin (methylphenidate) given intravenously or intramuscularly in a dose of 20 to 30 mg., repeated after 30 minutes if necessary, will overcome the depression of barbiturate or tranquilizer overdosage. However, it must be stressed that reliance on these drugs alone is inadequate and monitoring and supportive measures must continue unabated.

CONVULSIONS

Convulsions are characterized by rapid onset with central nervous system stimulation manifested as hyperpnea, forceful expiration, twitching of first the facial muscles and later those of the extremities and trunk, progressing to repetitive muscular spasm. The pupils dilate, pulse is rapid and blood pressure elevated. The duration may be only a few moments or much longer. The causes are varied and include carbon dioxide retention, hypoxia, drug toxicity or preexisting convulsive disorder.

Treatment includes discontinuing the procedure and anesthetic administration, giving oxygen, control of the patient for maintaining the airway, prevention of injury, and verbal reassurance. A short-acting barbiturate (Nembutal or Seconal) is given intravenously in a dose of 50 mg. After waiting for effect, repeat the dose once or twice as needed. Incremental intravenous administration is most controllable but, if no vein is available, give the barbiturate intramuscularly (for safety, doses should be smaller). Give only the least amount of barbiturate necessary to control the seizure since its potential respiratory depression would later be additive to that normally following the seizure.

VOMITING

During sedative management, vomiting is more annoying than dangerous but should not be treated lightly, since airway obstruction and aspiration are still potentially possible. Keeping the patient on an empty stomach before treatment will help, since vomiting will be less likely to occur and, if it does, will be only of clear fluid with no odor or solid matter. Maintaining as even a level of sedation as possible (particularly with nitrous oxide) tends to lessen the incidence.

Treatment consists of lowering the patient to a supine position and rotating the head to the side so that vomitus tends to pool in the cheek. The mouth and pharynx should be suctioned clean and oxygen given as this lessens the feeling of nausea. With light sedation, treatment can usually be resumed after a brief episode of vomiting.

VENIPUNCTURE SITE COMPLICATIONS

Traumatic Venipuncture

Insertion of a needle into a vein should always be done with careful technique in as gentle a manner as possible. Every step should be uncompromisingly followed, omitting nothing. Veins must be suitable: large enough, straight and accessible. The tourniquet should be applied tightly enough to block venous return, thereby engorging the veins and facilitating entry into them. The needle should be advanced only when the tourniquet is in place, with the bevel up and with an upward pressure on the point to help avoid further penetration of the vessel wall. Entry into a vein necessitates injuring its wall by puncturing it at some site, but this puncture can be kept small by advancing the needle decisively with a single thrust rather than by threading it back and forth (alternately advancing and withdrawing). The overlying skin must be adequately fixed and a rolling vein immobilized.

All of these steps are important, but even when they are scrupulously followed, a venipuncture site will occasionally evidence pain or a hematoma for a few days. Removal of the needle from the vein leaves a small hole through which some blood may exit to the enveloping tissues. Direct pressure with a gauze square for a few minutes (longer time for females) will help prevent internal hemorrhage. The patient should be reassured that a hematoma will disappear as does one resulting from other causes, and that resolution can be hastened by application of warm moist compresses.

Phlebitis

Inflammation of a vein, phlebitis, is rarely seen with good intravenous technique but does occasionally occur and is characterized by moderate pain, some edema, a hardened cordlike appearance of the affected vein segment and, possibly, some redness. The time before onset is variable from one day to as long as a week.

The potential causes for phlebitis include vein trauma, too frequent use of the same site, irritation by the needle during insertion, prolonged retention at the same site, or use of especially strong solutions. If the blood flow through the vein is slowed as a result of constriction of the arm by too tight fixation, the intravenous agent will remain at the site for too long a time. Many agents (particularly barbiturates and phenothiazines) are irritating and by remaining too long can cause pain and vessel spasm immediately and phlebitis later.

Pain and spasm can be eliminated by injection of 5 to 10 ml. of 1 percent Procaine around the venipuncture site to dilute and neutralize the solution while relieving pain and breaking the vessel spasm. Phlebitis is treated by application of moist heat three or four times daily until the area becomes asymptomatic. Butazolidin (phenylbutazone), a nonspecific anti-inflammatory agent, given orally in doses of 100 mg. three to four times per day for five days, helps relieve pain and swelling. This drug potentiates insulin and is contraindicated for patients on anticoagulants or those with peptic ulcer. Side effects such as nausea and edema are possible but rare with this type of management.

Extravasation of Agents

If blood escapes from the vein, a bluish swelling will develop around the site and a hematoma will form but if intravenous solutions or agents extravasate, the swelling will be colorless and some pain and tissue damage may result. If only dextrose solution escapes, the swelling is of lesser consequence as the solution is isotonic and not irritating.

No solution should be injected until it has been determined by testing for positive aspiration and dripping in some dextrose solution, seeing no swelling forms, and that the needle lumen is completely within the vein. Only dilute solutions should be used. Repeated injections should be made into the tubing of the intravenous infusion rather than into the vein. When the drug escapes from the vein it will have the effect of a subcutaneous injection rather than an intravenous one.

Whenever a swelling becomes evident, the drip should be stopped. A small swelling can be dispersed and damage prevented by massaging the area. Extravasation of larger volumes should be treated with warm, moist compresses. Pain in the area is treated by injection of 5 to 10 ml. of 1 percent procaine at the site. Medical consultation should be sought if there is necrosis, ulceration or discoloration of tissues.

Intra-arterial Injection

Entry into a superficial artery is rare but is more likely in the antecubital fossa than on the dorsum of the hand. The antecubital fossa is most often used as a venipuncture site since the veins there are larger and fixed (do not roll). Before a tourniquet is applied, the vessel should be palpated to assure absence of a pulse. If an artery is entered, the blood will be very bright red and will be ejected into the syringe much more forcefully than from a vein. (The plunger may actually be pushed back out of the syringe.) Also, the patient is apt to feel intense pain as the artery closes down in spasm and the forearm and hand distal to the site blanch quite noticeably. It is possible that some (or even all) of the signs may be absent, but if there is any doubt

no sedative drug should be injected into that site.

If proper technique is followed the initial injection of a drug will involve only a small test dose so that the sequelae, even after intra-arterial injection, will not be catastrophic. If the patient feels an intense, burning pain radiating down the arm from the injection site with, or without, blanching of the skin, the injection should be stopped immediately but *the needle should not be removed*. Then 10 ml. of 1 percent procaine should be injected directly into the artery to relieve the pain and relax the spasm. Medical consultation is imperative, since a brachial plexus or stellate ganglion block may be necessary to break the spasm. The pain is likely to be so intense as to make avoidance of recognition and treatment impossible but if remediation is delayed or inadequate there is a possibility of ischemic necrosis of tissue and, in the extreme, loss of fingers, hand or even the forearm because of gangrene.

Injection into a Nerve

Trauma to a nerve trunk may result in sensory or motor impairment. Prevention is essential and is accomplished by using only superficial veins that can be visualized when engorged after application of a tourniquet. Venipuncture should never be done blindly. While some experienced operators may claim that they can enter veins by feel alone, this is questionable and more likely to be bravado than tact and certainly not for inexperienced clinicians to attempt. Enter veins only in deliberate direct movements (preferably only a single thrust) and never probe with the needle to find a vein you cannot see.

Infection

Fortunately the vascular system is well equipped to fight infection and this is rare at a venipuncture site if the normal precepts of aseptic technique are followed. The injection site should be clean and swabbed with an antiseptic solution prior to insertion. Once you have swabbed the area do not touch it again. The skin and underlying tissues often must be fixed by digital pressure but the finger should be applied an inch or so away from the injection site, pulling the skin away from it. All armamentaria must be sterile. Disposable needles and syringes, in addition to saving time, are sterilized better than we can do so in our offices and are preferable to resterilized, reusable materials. The packages must, needless to say, be unbroken and all supplies should be used only once, with care to avoid contamination.

Defective Armamentarium

The commonly available disposable needles, syringes and infusion sets are of high quality and malfunction is rare. However, prudence dictates that all armamentaria should be tested (contamination being avoided) before use. The plunger in each syringe should be withdrawn and readvanced to test the syringe and patency of the needle. The needle point should be inspected. The infusion set should be allowed to run not only to expel air from the tubing but also to assure its proper function.

EMERGENCY SUPPLIES

Effective treatment of emergency situations requires not only know-how but also the immediate availability of certain supplies and drugs. A set of these supplies should be put aside, reserved only for emergency use, and not drawn upon for normal usage. This emergency kit must be instantly available and should be inspected frequently to be certain that nothing is missing or that the drugs contained therein are not outdated.

There are many drugs to serve any specific purpose, but for simplicity and efficiency only one for each therapeutic indication should be included in the emergency kit (one antihistamine, one narcotic antagonist, one corticosteroid, etc.).

APPARATUS

Oxygen (face mask, breathing bag)
Stethoscope
Sphygmomanometer
Mouth prop (McKesson rubber, Molt mechanical)
Suction tip
Disposable syringes—2, 5, 20 ml.
Disposable needles—18 ga. x 1½ in.
　　　　　　　　　　20 ga. x 1½ in.
　　　　　　　　　　22 ga. x 1½ in.
Tourniquet
Intravenous infusion sets
Alcohol swabs
Armboard
Tongue forceps
Tongue depressors
Cricothyrostomy cannula with trocar
Intracardial needle—22 ga. x 3½ in.
Airways—oropharyngeal—small, medium, large

DRUGS

Adrenalin (epinephrine)
Aminophylline
Ammonia pearl (aromatic ammonia spirit)
Amyl nitrite pearl
Atropine—1/150 gr. per ml.
Benadryl (diphenhydramine)
Dextrose 5% in water (500 ml. bottles)
Nalline (nalorphine)
Nembutal (pentobarbital)
Neosynephrine (phenylephrine)
Nitroglycerin (glyceryl trinitrate sublingual tablets)
Procaine 1%
Ritalin (methylphenidate)
Seconal (secobarbital)
Solu-Cortef (hydrocortisone)
Wyamine (mephentermine)

16 | Relation to Dental Operative Situations

By relaxing patients both mentally and physically, it is possible to make our procedures more acceptable and to complete them more effectively and with less effort. Both the patient and the doctor benefit, the former with better dental care and the latter with less fatigue and greater satisfaction.

With relaxation, lessened awareness of pain, some degree of amnesia and pleasant recovery, patients find that they no longer dread the prospect of dental treatment. As contrasted with general anesthetic management, these patients, being awake and suggestible, can be trained to accept dentistry, are often weaned from the more profound sedative methods, and will return for routine periodic recall examination submitting to treatment performed by more conventional means.

There are, of course, sedative failures; some patients can never be successfully treated in this manner. Rapport and communication are necessary. If these are lacking, as they might be with retarded or severely uncooperative patients, there may be no choice but re-referral for treatment with general anesthesia. These persons represent an exceedingly small percentage of the population.

Once a decision has been made to sedate a patient, there still must be a determination which method to use. The ideal is the least potent method that provides adequate operating conditions so that the patient's bodily functions and daily routine are upset as little as possible. With experience it is usually possible to improve the results obtained from any given regimen and to lessen the depth of sedation necessary to complete treatment.

When nitrous oxide analgesia is employed as the sole sedative regimen, the patient need not be accompanied or come with an empty stomach. With the rapid recovery usually obtained, he can safely leave the office alone. Further, with the machine kept handy in the treatment room, preoperative preparation is nil and the overall management often saves rather than costs time. Herein lies a major difference between nitrous oxide analgesia and the other sedative modalities; it can be considered normal treatment with no benefit to be derived from weaning patients from it. Further, treatment can be planned as for unsedated patients rather than for completion in one or only a few visits. For patients for whom deeper sedation is used, the weaning process can often be considered finished when they can be treated with analgesia (and local) alone. This will be the "normal" treatment method for this individual.

For profoundly fearful patients, for whom deeper sedation is needed, local anesthesia should always be used. With those for whom nitrous oxide analgesia is the sole sedation there is some leeway and various combinations of management are possible. The analgesia may be used only to mask the intra-

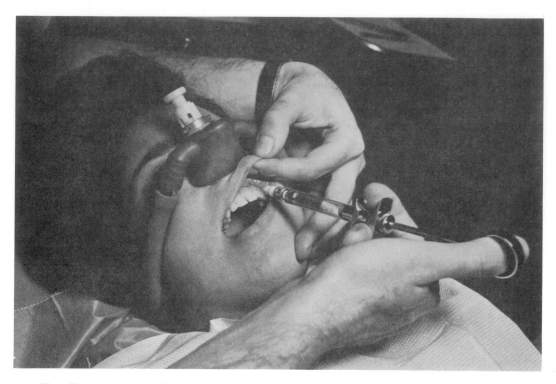

Fig. 56. Injection of a local anesthetic must be accomplished with all the care and finesse of similar injections on unsedated patients. The mask position and other aspects of the sedative situation interfere neither with access nor injection technique.

oral injections and then be terminated. Local may be used for only more painful procedures and not for others at a given session. The discomfort of numbness from bilateral mandibular blocks can be avoided, local being used for the less involved side while treatment is completed at one session, thus saving another appointment for that quadrant. Some procedures causing only mild discomfort (prophylaxis, seating and cementation of castings, dry-socket dressings, suture removal) can be accomplished with analgesia alone. By coordinating with local anesthetics, the duration of nitrous oxide administration can be shortened for nausea-prone patients.

Analgesia effectively eliminates the gagging often associated with radiography, impressions, tongue retraction or suctioning towards the pharynx. Since patients will cough up debris falling back into the pharynx, throat packs are not necessary. Objections to the noise or vibrations of the drill, the scraping of curettage or the pressure of luxation during extraction are minimized. With a lesser awareness of the passage of time, long appointments will be more pleasant. This phenomenon, plus the muscular relaxation, allows for maintenance of a mouth prop, facilitating access to posterior areas while eliminating interruptions as the patient closes his mouth. Similarly, many of the problems associated with acceptance of a rubber dam are avoided. Discomfort from water spray and suctioning is lessened. The use of electro-surgical apparatus or an open flame are not contraindicated.

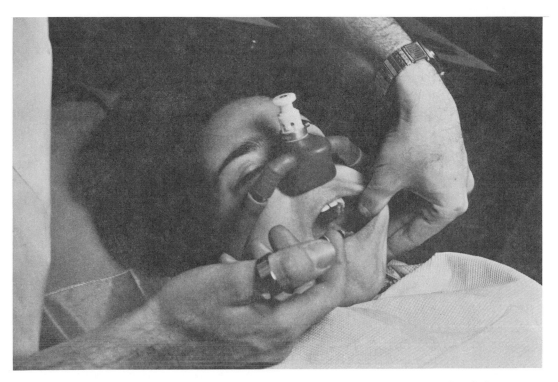

FIG. 57. With most sedation, the patient can cooperate by maintaining an open mouth. Our injection procedure proceeds the same as for the unsedated patient.

Safety is effectively attained by monitoring the patient's reactions with methods ranging from simple observation with analgesia to more detailed techniques for deeper sedation. It is possible to schedule long appointments in order to increase operative productivity without greatly disrupting the patient's daily routine.

TREATMENT PLANNING

The treatment plan and sedative regimen may be contingent upon the patient's physical status. A careful dental examination, while essential, is no more important than a thorough history, physical examination and medical consultation. Some relatively elective dental procedures may have to be foregone or postponed because the necessary sedative regimen may be contraindicated by some aspect of the medical profile.

Since, during sedative management, the patient will be in no position to discuss alternate treatment plans, he should be informed of questionable prognoses and of contingent treatment plans at the preoperative evaluation session. Doubtful undertakings should be avoided since, with the demands of sedative management, it may be impractical to schedule extra appointments to correct unsuccessful results. If the cavity is large, and if endodontic treatment, pin reinforcement or full coverage may be needed, inform the patient of this before treatment. Be certain that he understands that treatment will be completed in relatively few appointments and that the payment arrangements must reflect this. Finally, give your preoperative instructions (preferably in writing) as to empty stomach, accompanying adult, clothing, makeup, and so forth.

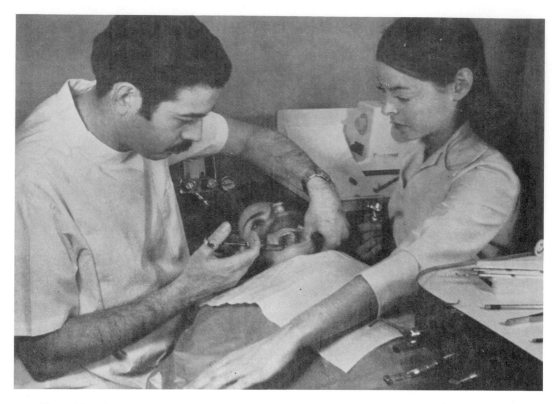

FIG. 58. Occasionally patients may react to injection with body or limb movements. The assistant's hand should hover across the patient's arms, ready to guide them but offering no restraining force.

Carefully plan the sequence of treatment, combining the various disciplines of dental practice for a single session (operative dentistry, endodontics, periodontics, and so on). Once you have anesthetized an area, do everything possible in that region. Think in terms of quadrants rather than of specific dental disciplines. Plan long appointments so that once sedation has been established, the maximum benefit can be derived; with the possible exception of nitrous oxide analgesia, the production of a sedated state takes time and the fewer times this is necessary the better will be the results. Prescribe or dispense any indicated premedicating agents. Finally, for the comfort of patients who have not eaten, schedule cases early in the day.

Before beginning, decide upon the type of sedation and the presumptive doses by considering physical status, age, suitability of veins, cooperativeness, depth required, length of the procedure and proneness to nausea. When making your daily schedule allow for any latent period before onset of sedative effect as well as for a recovery period. It is possible to treat another patient at these times but the procedures planned should be such as to allow you to observe the sedated patient occasionally. For efficiency it is essential that you have more than one treatment room.

OFFICE EQUIPMENT

While our office equipment should always be operating at peak efficiency,

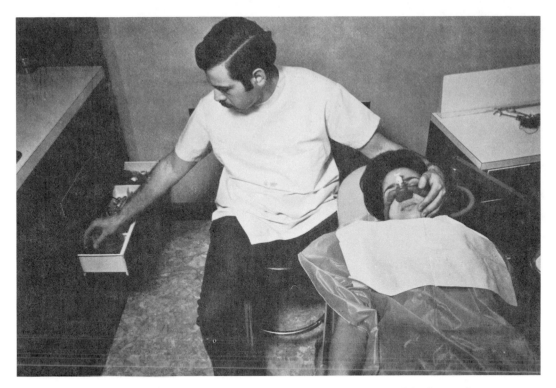

FIG. 59. To properly monitor it is essential that contact with the patient never be lost. When turning away, a hand on the face will monitor the state of relaxation, head position, skin temperature and moisture, mouth opening, movement and general situation of the patient.

this requirement is particularly important during sedative management. Interruptions for repair or replacement of defective equipment are most disconcerting. Handpieces should be cleaned and lubricated, water sprays should be adjusted etc. Adequate supplies of consumable items should be at hand. Each case should begin with new burs.

Injection supplies and monitoring equipment should be prepared and tested, syringes loaded, spare drugs be inconspicuously available. Tape, bandages, armboard and alcohol sponges, if they are to be used, should be within arm's reach. The anesthesia machine should be checked and a suitable mask attached. In summation, anything that might be needed, even if the need is rather remote, should be instantly available and ready for use.

APPLICATION TO SPECIFIC AREAS OF DENTAL PRACTICE

Operative Dentistry

The plan will vary with the nature and quantity of treatment required and the method of sedation. For some patients full mouth treatment will be accomplished at a single session; but for others, because of the magnitude, only half the mouth or a single quadrant will be completed. It is not always possible to complete a given area without returning to it again, but this should be our goal.

Since the production of most sedative states requires time at each session,

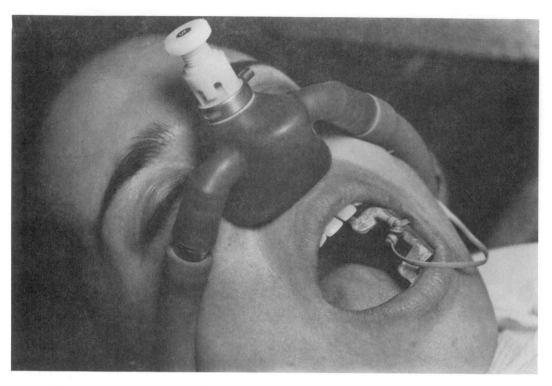

Fig. 60. The rubber McKesson mouth props, available in several sizes, can be used for either side.

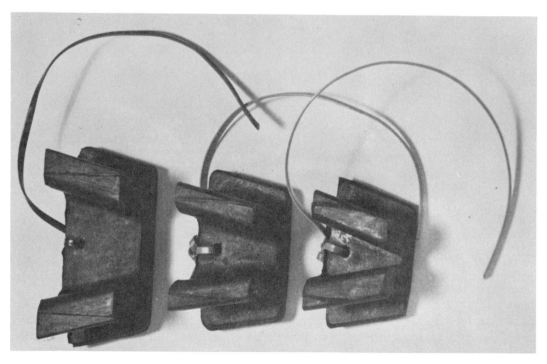

Fig. 61. Size comparison of the rubber McKesson mouth props. Place the prop so that the solid side is toward the cheek and the open side toward the tongue. A string sometimes aids in removal but is optional.

extensive treatment is most efficiently performed at long appointments. Sedated patients better accept this regimen and remain relaxed and cooperative for longer periods. In many cases the factors limiting the length of the session are more related to the operator's stamina than they are to the patient's responsiveness. Generally, patients accept most operative procedures well. They will not object to a water spray, high-velocity suction equipment, noise or vibration of drills, operative manipulation, cotton rolls or rubber dam. Any objection they do make is usually mild and easily managed. They lose awareness of the passage of time so that they can keep their mouths open for long periods (with the aid of a mouth prop if necessary), and this greatly improves our access and vision. Their desire to rinse disappears and with it go most of the interruptions.

Sedative management can take many forms. Understandably, shorter treatment plans often can be completed with lesser sedation. Patients may wish not to undergo deeply sedated treatment marathons, preferring more and shorter sessions under lighter sedation. Nitrous oxide analgesia, for most, represents the best mild to moderate sedation for sessions lasting under an hour. Patients need not be premedicated, accompanied, or be on an empty stomach. Local anesthesia can be used selectively; this is required for some situations and can be avoided in others. Many procedures if they are only mildly uncomfortable, can be done with analgesia alone (trial and cementation of castings, occlusal adjustment), thus allowing the patient to leave without aftereffects. Some can have virtually all of

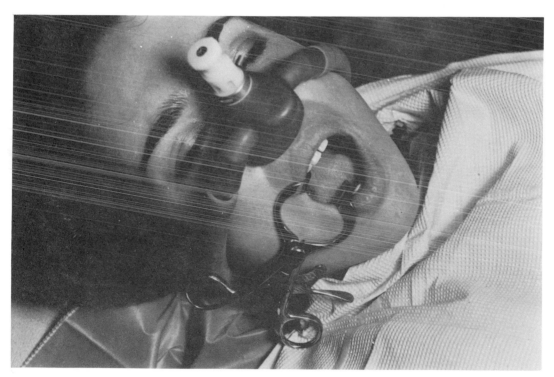

FIG. 62. The Molt mechanical mouth prop adjusts to various mouth opening positions. It does not occupy any space within the mouth but does not keep its position as reliably as do the intraoral props.

their treatment done under analgesia without local; others need local only for specific, more painful situations. Sedation can be carried deeper for procedures requiring it and then be lightened later as less disturbing facets are completed (e.g., deeper for crown preparation, lighter for impressions, bite registration, fabrication of temporary coverage).

Sedation is compatible with all our operative procedures and treatment methods complementing four-handed sit-down dentistry, requiring no compromises in restorative planning and interfering with none of our techniques or equipment.

Pedodontics

When children are introduced to dental treatment there is the ever-present possibility that an unsuccessful or unpleasant beginning will create a negative impression that will persist throughout life. Lifelong benefits are derived from pleasant introduction of dental treatment to children. The relaxed patient can be treated by a relaxed doctor.

With their vivid imaginations children are highly suggestible and particularly amenable to training (especially when their suggestibility is heightened by medication). Sedative masking of any unpleasantness aids in the establishment of a comfortable state and reinforces the feeling that dental treatment is a nonthreatening experience. Creation of a fantasy situation is a more effective means of suggestion in children than is the prediction of subjective symptoms (see analgesia induction techniques, p. 89).

Since their span of attention is short, children often benefit from the lack of awareness of the passage of time. Se-

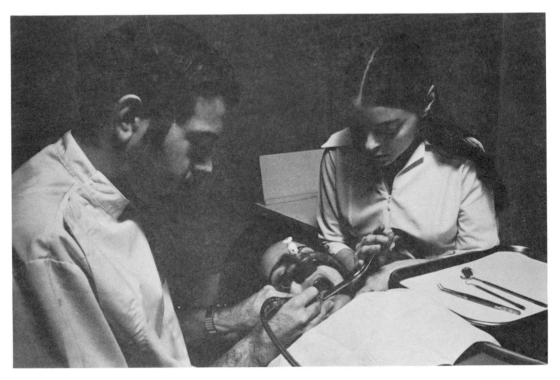

Fig. 63. Sedative management is compatible with four-handed sit-down dentistry and offers no contraindication to the use of ultraspeed equipment, water spray or high velocity suction equipment.

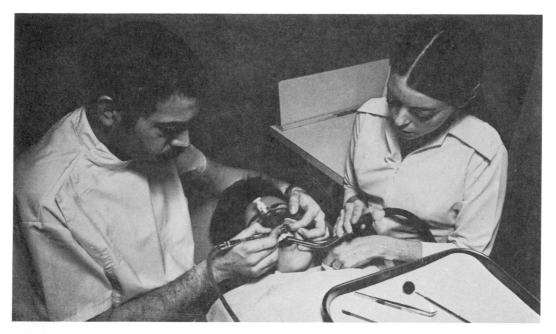

FIG. 64. Operative access is not limited by the presence of a nasal mask. The soft rubber masks, particularly, maintain their seal against the skin, preventing leakage of gases even though the lips and cheeks are widely retracted.

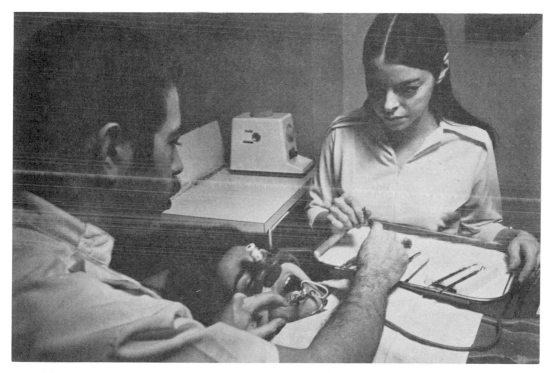

FIG. 65. Efficient operating procedures, while valuable for all treatment, are especially beneficial during sedative management.

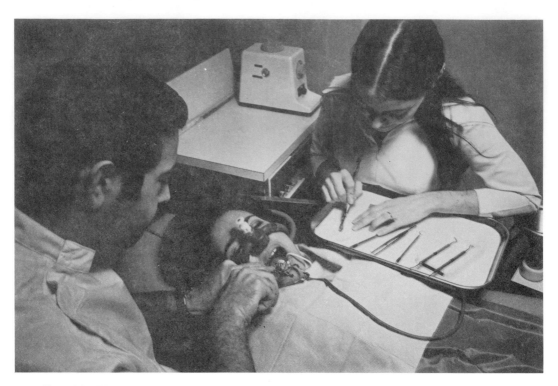

Fɪɢ. 66. Most operative procedures can be accomplished in the same manner as for nonsedated patients. The supine position, needed in deeper sedation to prevent postural hypotension, is the position used for sit-down dentistry.

dative quiescence lessens movement of the trunk, limbs or tongue and expedites treatment. A rubber dam, so often used in pedodontics, is compatible with sedative management. The lessened mouth breathing increases the inhalation of nitrous oxide and enhances the efficacy of analgesia. However, since there is less air dilution the inspired concentration of nitrous oxide must usually be reduced.

The strange feeling of numbness from local anesthesia, never before experienced, may be frightening to some children, and if this can be avoided a positive benefit accrues. The numbness may be incorrectly interpreted by a child as pain and it is difficult to explain to him that this is not so. Further, children often cause postoperative discomfort by biting their cheeks, lips or tongue.

Many cavities in deciduous teeth can be filled by using only nitrous oxide analgesia without local. This modality is also sufficiently analgesic to extract loose deciduous teeth. If local must be used, its effects can be confined to smaller areas. Radiography or full mouth impressions can be rendered less disturbing when the child is sedated. If the impression or the radiographs are the sole procedure, the rapid in-and-out sedation of analgesia is best.

Sedation of an extremely uncooperative child is often impossible, and a general anesthetic must be used. Intramuscular injection may be indicated in some children who refuse oral medication. The gluteal area presents probably the best injection site, since it allows for more efficient immobilization of the child during the injection (see intramuscular injection technique, p.

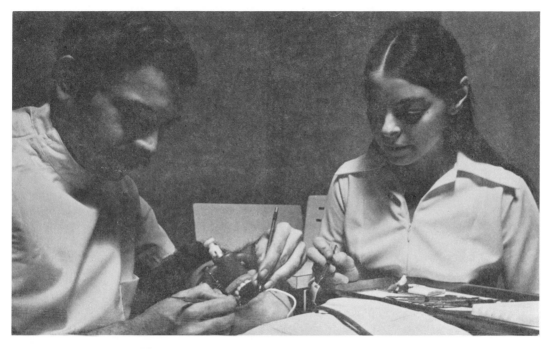

Fig. 67. The nasal mask does not interfere with visual access to the mouth whether by direct or indirect vision.

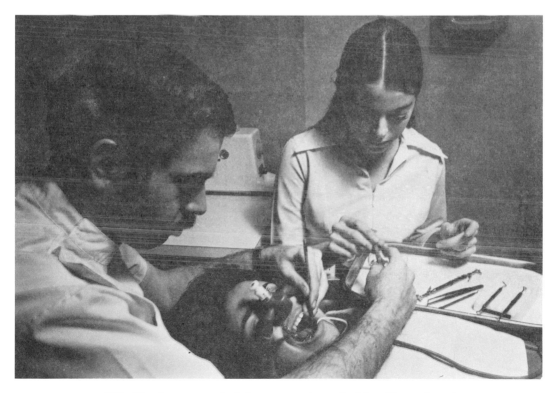

Fig. 68. Access and vision are unimpeded in all quadrants.

117). Analgesia induction is often unsuccessful for the child who is crying or screaming, since each outcry is accompanied by a gulp of air that may excessively dilute the inspired gas mixture. Also, some children are chronic mouth breathers so, for them, inhalation is a less effective route of administration than the others. Oral premedication is more effective when given at home than when it is given in the office. In some cases a basal level of sedation in this manner will render the child more amenable to the nasal mask

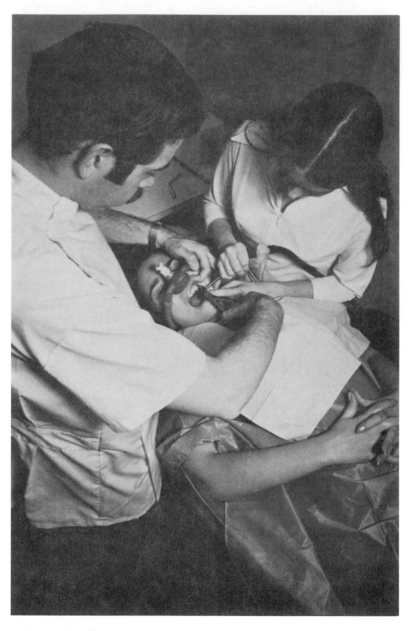

FIG. 69. The excellent skin adaptation of the soft nasal masks allows for adequate access and vision for surgical procedures.

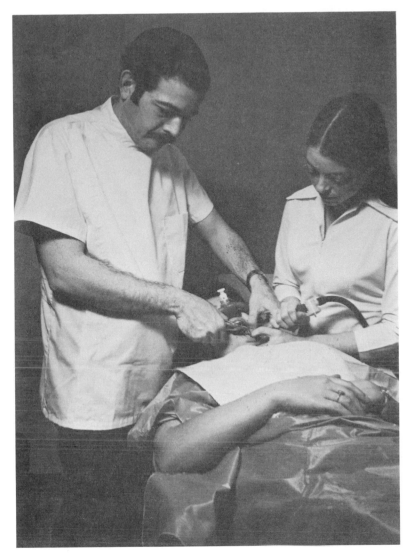

Fig. 70. Procedures better performed by a standing operator should be accomplished by raising the chair while keeping the patient in the same supine position as for sit-down dentistry.

and will allow for more effective nasal breathing so that analgesia will become the method of choice. In any case, injection of an intraoral local anesthetic will be better tolerated by a sedated patient.

Oral Surgery

Surgical procedures of any type are particularly frightening to most pa-

tients. Some who are quite able to take most dental procedures in stride require some form of sedation for surgery. With effective sedation, general anesthesia can usually be avoided but local anesthesia is always mandatory.

Sedation aids the patient in keeping his mouth open for extended periods and in accepting a mouth prop which may be necessary if mouth opening is

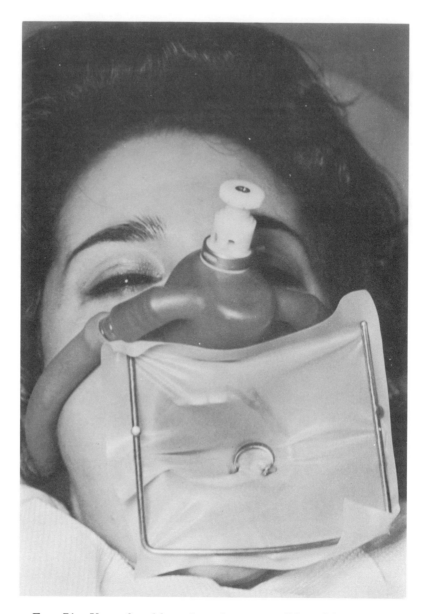

FIG. 71. Use of rubber dam is compatible with the nasal mask. Since the air dilution of mouth breathing is reduced, the inhaling valve should be opened or the concentration of nitrous oxide reduced.

to be wide enough for access to posterior regions. The sight of blood or surgical instruments, the pressure of luxation, the pounding of a chisel or the scraping of a curette or bone file are less objectionable to a sedated patient. Hemostasis is aided by use of epinephrine-containing local anesthetic solutions which are not contraindicated as they are with some general anesthetic agents.

Choice of sedative modality depends largely upon the surgical procedure contemplated. Intramuscular or intra-

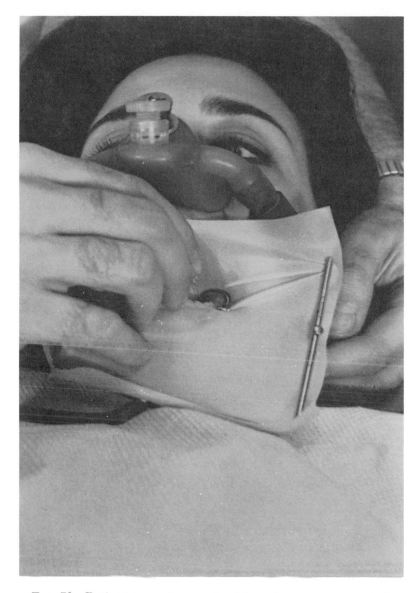

Fig. 72. Patient acceptance of rubber dam, open mouth for extended periods and the tedium of root canal instrumentation are enhanced by sedative muscular relaxation and lessening of time awareness.

venous sedation would be quite inefficient for a single extraction. The sedation would be a greater undertaking than the surgery and the length of the recovery period would be unacceptable. Nitrous oxide analgesia is, by far, the method of choice. On the other hand, analgesia would probably not be best as the sole sedation for lengthier procedures such as removal of an impacted third molar, apicoectomy or periodontoplasty.

Analgesia may suffice as the only medication for mildly painful peripheral procedures such as suture removal, dry-socket dressing, irrigation under an inflamed pericoronal flap or a dressing change. It may also add the necessary analgesic potency when the local anesthetic is not quite effective enough. Oxygen in the inspired mixture is not incompatible with electrosurgery. Gagging from tongue retraction, third molar radiography, mouth prop or suction in the pharynx will be eliminated. A small-sized flexible nasal mask will not hinder access to the gingival areas even above the maxillary incisors (as is necessary for apicoectomy or frenectomy).

Endodontics

While sedation may be helpful, extirpation of a vital pulp can be performed on an awake patient only with effective local anesthesia. The tedium of prolonged endodontic therapy will be less objectionable to a sedated patient as will be the perception of uncomfortable proprioceptive stimuli caused by instrumentation of a canal or condensation of a filling.

A rubber dam is often uncomfortable because of inability to swallow or to close the mouth. Analgesia can be used but, since mouth breathing is lessened, the concentration of nitrous oxide should be decreased and the inhaling valve opened. It is ideal, also, for short procedures which require little anesthesia such as gaining access to a hot chamber or clearing debris from a clogged tooth that had been left open for drainage. Electrosterilization of a

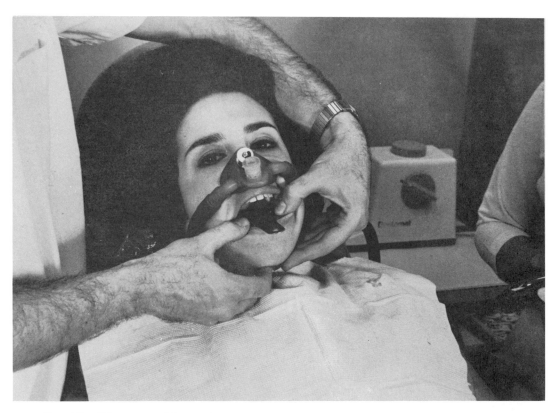

FIG. 73. Nitrous oxide analgesia provides excellent sedation for taking impressions. Since postural hypotension is not a problem, the patient may be seated upright.

canal or use of an open flame with gutta-percha are not contraindicated by the presence of oxygen.

Sedation administered orally or by injection is usually best for long sessions (especially endodontic surgical procedures) but analgesia may also be beneficial. With the use of a small, flexible nasal mask, adequate access and vision are obtained even for apicoectomy on the maxillary incisors. The soft masks can maintain their seal against the skin even when the upper lip is retracted.

Prosthodontics

Prosthetic dentistry involves a host of procedures that can be hindered by a jittery or tense patient. Registration of occlusal relationships is facilitated by relaxed musculature, since patients will more readily follow instructions and accept guidance. Local anesthetic interference with proprioceptive sensation often hinders accurate centric registration. Sedation, making prolonged, tedious appointments less objectionable, also eliminates the need for local anesthetic for many situations. The sedative regimen can be tailored to the needs of the moment (deeper for major tooth reductions, lighter for impressions, occlusal adjustment or esthetic evaluation).

In removable prosthodontics there is seldom a need for sedation that is profound or of long duration. Mild sedation can be produced with oral administration and supplemented, as needed, for short periods with analgesia. Gagging on full-mouth impressions can be eliminated. Registration of muscle borders need not be hindered by the nasal mask, as the softer masks can be ap-

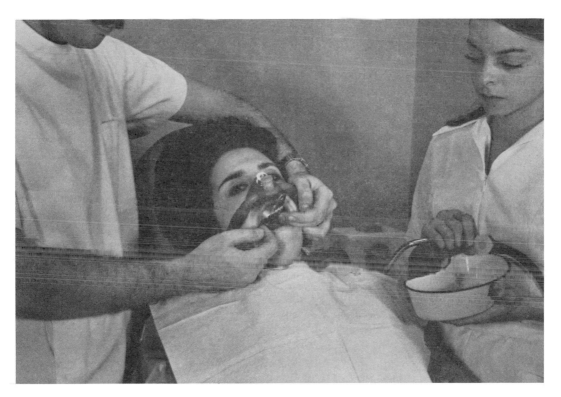

Fig. 74. Nitrous oxide analgesia virtually eliminates gagging during impressions. Registration of muscle borders is not hindered by the nasal mask.

plied somewhat loosely and manipulated without losing their seal against the skin. The objection to the taste and burning sensation of reline acrylic can be minimized. An open flame can be used to soften waxes or modeling compound. Rest seats are usually prepared and teeth are shaped without discomfort (even without local anesthesia).

Preprosthetic surgical procedures (frenectomy, muscle reattachment, ridge reduction and extension, torus removal) usually are better with the more profound sedation techniques. Local anesthesia is, of course, mandatory. Immediate denture insertion is best accomplished with deeper sedation during extraction with lighter levels for adjustment of the denture. The control inherent in intravenous administration facilitates this type of management but a single intramuscular injection at the beginning of the session can be successful too, as the sedation lightens while the case continues and the drug effect wanes.

Fixed prosthodontic procedures often require long appointments for crown preparations and impressions. Sedated patients accept more readily prolonged periods of airotor noise, water spray, suction and wide-open mouth and will be less disturbed by the odor of electrosurgical gingival retraction or the thermal shock of hydrocolloid. The access achieved through use of a mouth prop speeds crown preparations, particularly in the posterior areas. Relaxation of the patient increases the ability of the doctor by making long appointments easier. Analgesia lessens discomfort from seating and cementation of castings, occlusal adjustment (of teeth and castings) and removal of excess

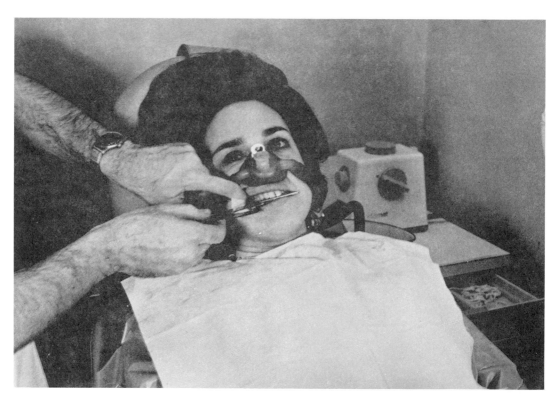

FIG. 75. Light sedation does not significantly interfere with proprioception so that occlusal registrations are valid. In fact, sedative muscular relaxation may aid in establishing and recording jaw relations.

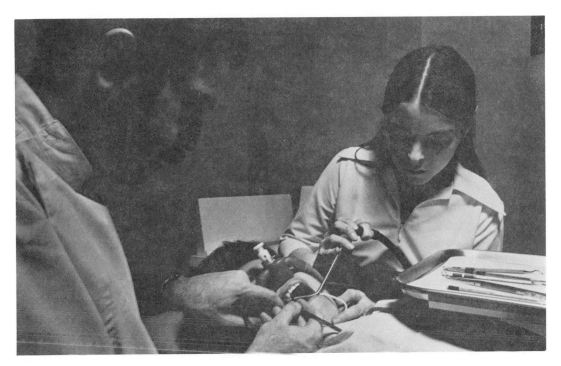

Fig. 76. Periodontal curettage can often be comfortably done on sedated patients without the need for local anesthetics. In such cases there is no limitation to any specific quadrant or area and the operator can range over the entire mouth.

cement, thus eliminating the need for local anesthesia which can be especially objectionable at widely dispersed areas.

Periodontics

With the use of analgesia, the patient can be spared the discomfort of gingival curettage or planing of hypersensitive root or cervical surfaces yet he can be alert enough immediately afterward to benefit from home care instruction and practice. Analgesia is especially beneficial, as its effects allow entry into all areas of the mouth at a single session and the tedium often associated with periodontal procedures is eliminated. It can facilitate, also, occlusal adjustment, shaping of teeth, elimination of overhanging margins and pack changes.

Deeper sedation (given intramuscularly or intravenously) will usually be indicated for surgical procedures with the method of sedation chosen according to the needs of the situation. Access is improved by wide mouth opening and relaxed musculature that allow lip, cheek and tongue retraction. Hemostasis is improved through the use of local anesthetic solutions containing epinephrine.

Orthodontics

The indications for sedation in orthodontics are limited, but they do exist. Usually the sedation is mild and is administered orally, but the other routes also can be beneficial. It would probably be impractical for a dentist in limited orthodontic practice to acquire an inhalation analgesia capability, but the general dentist may occasionally benefit by applying his sedative capability to the orthodontic treatment he may provide. Nitrous oxide analgesia would make more easy the acceptance of a

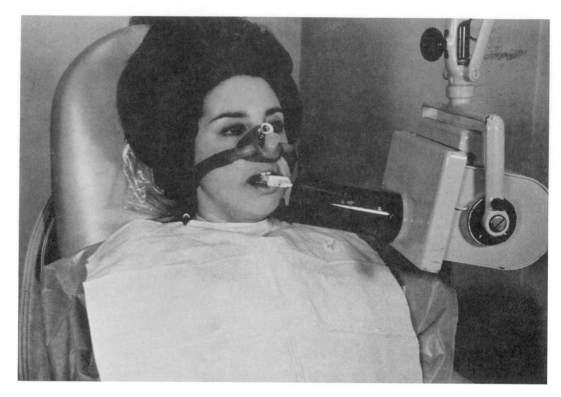

FIG. 77. Light sedation allows the patient to be seated upright and to cooperate in the taking of radiographs. Normal positioning and angulations are used without modification. With nitrous oxide analgesia, gagging is virtually eliminated.

number of orthodontic procedures such as seating of bands and removal of excess cement subgingivally, stripping of teeth and taking of full arch impressions.

Most orthodontic patients, being young, have relatively short attention spans and would benefit from mild sedation at a lengthy appointment intended for involved fixed appliance insertion. Measures employed to avoid moisture contamination of cement will be less bothersome and when the patient is more calm, salivary flow is somewhat diminished.

Radiography

As mentioned before, light levels of nitrous oxide analgesia virtually eliminate gagging on intraoral x-ray films in all cases and in all areas of the mouth. Patients are fully able to cooperate by opening and closing their mouths, maintaining head position as instructed and can hold the films. Since postural hypotension is not a problem, the chair can be adjusted to any position normally used for radiography; the patient can be fully upright. The newer soft rubber or plastic nasal masks and tubing are radiolucent; no special procedure need be followed in placing films or aiming the cone. Since full recovery is so rapid and since no special preoperative conditions need be met, analgesia can be used for radiography at any moment the need becomes apparent.

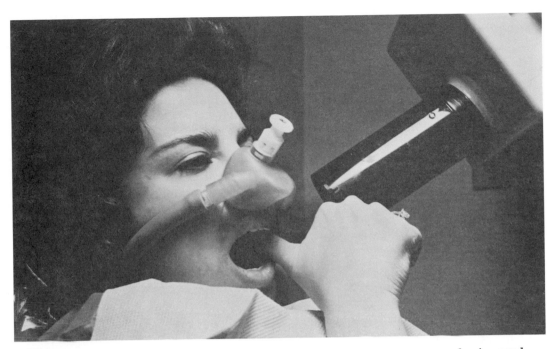

FIG. 78. Most nasal masks are radiolucent and their presence can be ignored while taking films.

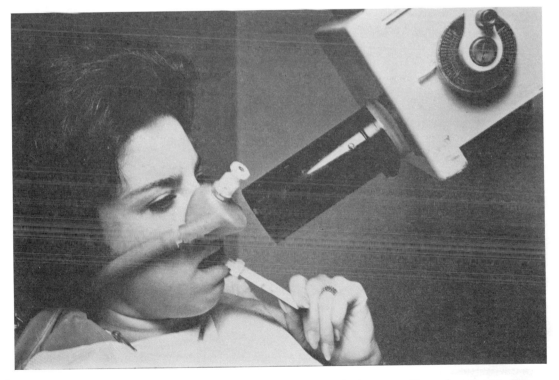

FIG. 79. The operator's preference in x-ray technique or film placement can be followed without change.

17 | General Anesthesia

The term general anesthesia describes a state of drug-induced unconsciousness characterized by obtundation of certain physiological responses. Induction into this state involves passage through the stages of analgesia and excitement and entrance into a third stage of surgical anesthesia which begins at the onset of automatic, regular respiration and continues to the point of cessation of spontaneous respiration from pharmacological paralysis of the respiratory centers in the central nervous system.

SPECIFIC REQUIREMENTS FOR MANAGEMENT

During general anesthesia various of the homeostatic mechanisms regulating vital functions are depressed and the patient must be carefully monitored so that derangements can be detected and appropriate remedial action undertaken. Trained personnel, medication and equipment to treat these occurrences must be instantly available.

Soft tissue relaxation may result in loss of airway following a falling-in of the walls of the respiratory passages and tongue or improper head position resulting from loss of tone in the muscles of the neck. Airway patency is sometimes insured by insertion of a tube through the larynx, between the vocal cords and into the trachea (endotracheal intubation).

Dental treatment almost invariably involves the presence of small particles of debris (crumbs of amalgam, wedges, tooth fragments, and so on) in the mouth. This is not dangerous for the awake patient who can gag and cough up these particles but while he is under general anesthesia these reflexes are absent and there is a real danger of aspiration and subsequent pulmonary pathology. Endotracheal intubation is especially indicated during dental treat-

ment because the presence of the tube can prevent entrance of particles into the trachea and lungs.

Vomiting cannot occur while a patient is maintained in the stage of surgical anesthesia but it can, and does, sometimes occur during induction or recovery at a time when the laryngeal reflex is absent and aspiration of vomitus may result. The methods for management of this eventuality should be known to any practitioner attempting general anesthesia.

Laryngospasm (loss of airway from a closing of the vocal cords), an occasional occurrence during induction or recovery, can cause death from suffocation as effectively as a garrote tightened around the neck. Treatment consists of breaking the muscular spasm in the vocal cords by administration of muscle-relaxant drugs, sometimes followed by endotracheal intubation. An alternate method, used by first-aiders rather than by anesthesiologists, involves performance of a cricothyrostomy, opening into the neck, and establishing an airway in this manner.

Management of general anesthesia is a procedure of sufficient complexity to preclude learning it from a text. Proficiency with this modality can come only from supervised administration of many anesthetics. This chapter is included only as background material to aid in providing a perspective against which to view sedative techniques and is not intended for implementation.

AGENTS—MODES OF ADMINISTRATION

Safe general anesthetic management, involving potent drugs, requires such fine control that only the intravenous or inhalation routes are used, with the other means of administration being reserved for preanesthetic or postoperative medication.

Intravenous administration involves use of the ultrashort-acting barbiturates which are noted to have an extremely pleasant and rapid induction but which serve poorly when used as the sole anesthetic for lengthy cases. Inhalation anesthetics are better for longer cases but have longer induction periods so that most often, in adults who do not object to venipuncture before induction of the anesthetic, intravenous methods are used for induction and then a switch is made to inhalation for maintenance. For children, inhalational agents are usually used throughout. Whatever the agent or mode of administration, the result is the same general anesthesia, exhibiting the same physiological responses and requiring basically the same type of management.

Intravenous

The three agents most commonly used for general anesthesia are Pentothal (thiopental sodium) and Surital (thiamylal sodium), both thiobarbiturates, and Brevital (methohexital sodium), a methylated oxybarbiturate. In our dental, ambulatory, outpatient treatment, Brevital is used most commonly, as it produces a more rapid, clearheaded recovery, but all three are

acceptable and exhibit similar anesthetic phenomena.

Barbiturates are not true anesthetics, since they are not analgesic and loss of consciousness is their major effect on the central nervous system. In subhypnotic doses, as in sedative management, there actually may be a relative lowering of the pain threshold. The sleep produced, not unlike dreamless natural sleep, does not prevent reaction to painful stimuli until the patient is depressed to an excessively deep level so that other agents should be used concomitantly for production of analgesia. Muscular relaxation similarly is not obtained until a state in which the medullary centers controlling respiration and circulation are markedly depressed. If profound relaxation is required, muscle-relaxant drugs should be used or the patient be switched to other anesthetics.

Intravenous barbiturates are well suited for use in dental offices as they are nonflammable and nonexplosive and postanesthetic nausea is rare. In short cases, as for a single extraction, recovery time to ambulation is very rapid and the patient can soon be discharged even though the rate of drug metabolization is only about 10 to 15 percent per hour. The rapid recovery, particularly with Brevital, is due to redistribution to such nonsensitive tissues as muscle and fat. After prolonged maintenance even Brevital produces slow recovery, as the reservoirs will be saturated and the redistribution mechanism can no longer function. The detoxification of the ultrashort-acting barbiturates occurs almost exclusively in the liver, contraindicating their use in patients with compromised liver function, for with these persons narcosis can be excessively prolonged.

The ultrashort-acting barbiturates are destroyed by gastric acidity and can be administered only intravenously. This contributes to their controllability (although never approaching that of inhalation agents because metabolization is necessary) but introduces certain difficulties as well. Venipuncture is required before induction but, whether because of inaccessible veins or noncooperation of the patient, this may not always be possible. The aqueous solutions of the barbiturates are extremely alkaline (pH greater than 10) and if extravasation should occur there is a possibility of pain, phlebitis, fibrosis or necrosis of the subcutaneous tissues.

Barbiturates depress the sensitivity of the respiratory center to carbon dioxide and lack the respiratory stimulating irritant effect of some inhalational general anesthetics, thereby causing a reduction of rate and depth of respiration. This effect, being related to dosage, is not marked after the subhypnotic doses of sedative management, but with general anesthesia can result in hypoventilation or apnea.

There tends to be some myocardial depression proportional to the amount of drug in contact with the heart and, in patients with poor cardiovascular reserve, this may constitute a serious problem. For any patient, the carbon dioxide retention accompanying hypoventilation may predispose to some cardiac arrhythmia, and lowered blood pressure may result from large doses.

The classic Guedel stages are not seen during barbiturate induction, because it proceeds so rapidly. While the dangers of passage through the excitement stage are avoided, there remains a relative sensitization of the laryngeal reflexes that may precipitate laryngospasm or bronchospasm. Local stimulation such as that caused by blood, mucus or particles should be avoided by suctioning the offending

substances and active bronchial asthmatic patients should be spared barbiturate anesthesia. The hiccoughing that often accompanies Brevital anesthesia is due to a different mechanism (stimulation of the phrenic nerve to the diaphram) and is of concern more because of interference with the operative procedure than for any danger to the patient.

Inhalation

Because they are inert in the body and rapidly excreted unchanged by the lungs (except Trilene), inhalation agents offer the greatest controllability of any general anesthetics. Varying the arterial tension by changing the inhaled concentration or by "washing out" with oxygen will alter the concentration in the brain as we desire without delayed effect from accumulation of breakdown products.

The inhalation agents are complete anesthetics in that they possess analgesic properties (block transmission of impulses from the periphery to the higher centers) in addition to having the ability to produce hypnosis and profound relaxation.

While respiratory depression may accompany administration it tends to be less profound than that seen with barbiturate anesthesia, because with diminished tidal volume less anesthetic vapor will be inspired (a somewhat self-limiting mechanism) and also because ventilation may be augmented by activation of local lung reflexes which result from contact with the anesthetic vapors.

Induction, not requiring venipuncture, can be accomplished even with the most uncooperative patients. Since hypnosis occurs more slowly, the classic Guedel stages and signs of anesthesia are seen to some degree and may aid in determination of anesthetic depth.

Nitrous Oxide

Nitrous oxide is the workhorse of anesthetics, being included in virtually every management regardless of what other agents are included. It is mildly hypnotic and analgesic and produces these effects independently of hypoxia which, should it occur, would produce effects which are additive. The margin of safety with nitrous oxide is great, danger being associated with hypoxia of incorrect usage.

The major disadvantage of nitrous oxide is its lack of potency. Surgical anesthesia of the first plane, if it can be obtained without hypoxically curtailing the oxygen flow, is approached after only a long induction and requires premedicants or adjuvant anesthetics for its maintenance. In the absence of hypoxia, the respiratory, vasomotor, vomiting and vagus centers are not affected so vital signs remain stable. Since metabolization is not necessary and excretion occurs through the lungs, liver or kidney pathology do not necessarily contraindicate nitrous oxide anesthesia. Aided by more potent analgesics, it can be used for high-risk patients.

Fluothane (Halothane)

An extremely potent anesthetic, halothane, is probably the most usual agent in dental offices because of its very rapid, smooth induction and recovery characteristics as well as its nonflammability and despite the fact that its use requires precision-calibrated heat-compensated vaporizers.

Depression of the myocardium can lead to decreased cardiac output, bradycardia and, during deep anesthesia, arrhythmias (particularly ventricular extrasystoles). Bradycardia, most commonly seen during induction of children, could conceivably progress to cardiac arrest. Blood pressure drop, varying with inspired concentration, tends to be greater during induction than during maintenance. Concomitant use of epinephrine or other pressor amines may lead to arrhythmia and is contraindicated.

During deep anesthesia the respiratory center is depressed with the potential for respiratory arrest (fortunately, preceding cardiac arrest), but during maintenance at the lighter levels usually indicated, respiratory depression is more likely to be the product of premedicants rather than of halothane.

Irritation of the respiratory mucosa is slight; coughing and secretions are not notably stimulated and the bronchi are not especially prone to spasm. Muscular relaxation is adequate for major surgery.

There has been much controversy as to potential liver toxicity as the cause of hepatic necrosis and this question has yet to be adequately resolved.

Penthrane (Methoxyflurane)

A potent, relatively new, anesthetic capable of producing surgical anesthesia without recourse to other agents, methoxyflurane possesses a low vapor pressure that eliminates the need for elaborate vaporizers required for halothane and adds a factor of safety to its administration. Induction and recovery are longer than those seen with halothane, with the postanesthetic period characterized by a hangover analgesic effect that may obviate or reduce the need for pain-allaying drugs for several hours.

The potential for cardiovascular stability is noteworthy; blood pressure remains within normal limits after the induction period and cardiac rhythm (in the absence of carbon dioxide retention) tends to remain free of arrhythmias even if epinephrine must be used.

Respiration may be depressed during deeper anesthesia, with indication occasionally for manual assistance of ventilation.

Methoxyflurane does not stimulate secretions, is neither larnygospasmogenic nor bronchospasmogenic, and produces early and profound muscular relaxation; it is compatible with the muscle-relaxant drugs.

There may be some evidence of the Guedel signs (even though pupillary contraction and eye fixation usually continue throughout the case) but, as with halothane, monitoring the vital signs provides a more reliable assessment of the patient's status.

Ether (Diethyl Ether)

An extremely flammable agent, ether usage requires special conductive shoes, grounded anesthetic equipment and specially shielded electrical equipment, contraindicating its use in dental offices. Induction, particularly the excitement stage, tends to be a long, slow process and recovery is prolonged and noted for the high incidence of nausea. Due to its irritating qualities, ether stimulates the production of copious amounts of secretions.

Respiration is stimulated during light anesthesia, and blood pressure, which usually falls only in deep anesthesia, may be depressed at even lighter levels in elderly persons or those suffering from myocardial disease. Muscle relaxation is good and the bronchioles are dilated which renders this a good agent for asthmatics.

The Guedel signs, originally postulated for ether anesthesia, remain particularly valid but may be masked to some degree by premedicants.

Trilene (Trichlorethylene)

Unique among inhalation agents, a portion of the inhaled trichlorethylene is metabolized in the body. When used with nitrous oxide, the analgesia stage can be produced and maintained but induction to surgical levels of anesthesia is slow (only lighter levels are obtainable) and recovery tends to be prolonged.

Trichlorethylene is nonexplosive and nonflammable under clinical conditions, has a rather sweetish odor that is not unpleasant, does not stimulate salivary secretions to any significant degree, and seems, in normal use, to be free of liver pathology. The frequency with which nausea and vomiting occur is significant.

Cardiac arrhythmias which can occur during deep trichlorethylene anesthesia are usually characterized by auricular extrasystoles, but with the potential for ventricular tachycardia which may be a precursor to ventricular fibrillation. Concomitant use of epinephrine or most other vasopressors is contraindicated because of increased tendency to arrhythmia. Respiration, particularly its rate, is increased during light anesthesia.

Muscle-Relaxant Drugs

Passage of an impulse along a nerve's surface membrane results in a wave of depolarization and liberation of acetylcholine at the end plate. Acetylcholine at the myoneural junction prevents repolarization and permits the muscle to continue in a relaxed state.

Muscular relaxation for anesthetic purposes is produced in either of two ways, depending upon the type of drug used. The depolarizing agents (succinylcholine, diacetylcholine) produce an acetylcholine-like action; and as long as a sufficient amount of drug remains at the myoneural junction, the surface membrane of the nerve maintains its depolarized state and paralysis results.

The nerve-blocking or nondepolarizing agents (d-tubocurarine, gallamine, dimethyltubocurarine) prevent acetylcholine from reaching the receptor areas of the muscle cell membrane. The action of the chemical transmitter is blocked through combination of the blocking agent with receptors usually occupied by acetylcholine.

While muscle relaxation can be produced by deepening the anesthesia, profound relaxation is not usually obtained in this manner since the depth required would be accompanied by excessive depression of the vital functions. With relaxant drugs, skeletal muscles can be relaxed to a point of total flaccid paralysis while anesthesia is maintained at relatively uncomplicated lighter levels, thus avoiding greater depression and not prolonging recovery time. Laryngoscopic exposure of the vocal cords and placement of an endotracheal tube between them are greatly simplified by paralysis with a short-acting muscle relaxant such as succinylcholine (Anectine, Quelicin, Sucostrin) the effect of which is profound but only of three to five minutes' duration after a single paralyzing dose.

Smooth and cardiac muscles remain unaffected but skeletal muscle action and tone can be totally eliminated for the duration of drug effect, rendering the patient totally incapable of breathing and requiring artificial ventilation.

Endotracheal Intubation

Essential not only to the maintenance of general anesthesia but also to life itself is a patent airway. Intubation represents only a mechanical means of assuring this airway and is not an anesthetic technique in itself. It is the level of anesthesia produced, and not the means employed to attain it, that determines the indication for intubation. In order to tolerate a tube the patient must be sufficiently anesthetized for the laryngeal reflex to be obtunded.

The tube, after insertion through either the nose or mouth, is passed down the pharynx and then through the larynx between the vocal cords and into the trachea. According to the preference of the anesthesiologist or the needs of the situation, the patient may be awake or asleep, breathing spontaneously or paralyzed at intubation. The cords can be visualized through a laryngoscope or approached blindly by gauging the position of the tube by the amplitude of the breath sounds heard through it. Injury to the vocal cords is avoided by passing the tube while the cords are parted, either because of paralytic relaxation of the musculature or of normal inspiratory effort.

The benefits of intubation include assurance of airway patency regardless of head or body position, facilitation of secretion removal from the tracheobronchial tree, prevention of aspiration of particles or blood, reduction of dead space (the nasal cavity, mouth and pharynx are separated from the airway while the tube is in place), enhancement of control over respiration since leakage can be eliminated and positive pressure can be more reliably applied, and provision for the anesthesiologist to move some distance from the patient (away from interference with the operative field) without relinquishing his control.

There are some negative aspects of intubation as well, and these include possibility of increased resistance to breathing through a narrow tube or angulated adaptors, coughing or "bucking" on the tube if the level of anesthesia is too light, injury to the nasal mucosa, vocal cords or the tracheal walls resulting in nosebleed, postoperative hoarseness or sore throat, edema or infection of the larynx or trachea, or ulceration of the tracheal mucous membrane. There is also the possibility of insertion of the tube into the esophagus or production of laryngospasm while the tube is being placed or subsequently removed.

For dental treatment, which is rather unique in that the operative site is situated within the airway, endotracheal intubation is particularly beneficial but, in view of the possible untoward sequelae, this technique should be employed only by those sufficiently trained in its use.

Index